Virtual Clinical Excursions—Obstetrics-Pediatrics

for

McKinney, James, Murray, Nelson, and Ashwill:
Maternal-Child Nursing,
Fourth Edition

Virtual Clinical Excursions—Obstetrics-Pediatrics

for

McKinney, James, Murray, Nelson, and Ashwill:
Maternal-Child Nursing,
Fourth Edition

prepared by

Kelly Ann Crum, MSN, RN
Associate Faculty
Curriculum Development/Maternal Child Nursing Specialty
Health Sciences and Nursing Department
University of Phoenix, Online
Phoenix, Arizona

software developed by

Wolfsong Informatics, LLC
Tucson, Arizona

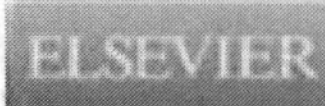

ELSEVIER
SAUNDERS

3251 Riverport Lane
Maryland Heights, Missouri 63043

VIRTUAL CLINICAL EXCURSIONS—OBSTETRICS-PEDIATRICS FOR MCKINNEY, JAMES, MURRAY, NELSON, AND ASHWILL: MATERNAL-CHILD NURSING
FOURTH EDITION

ISBN: 978-0-323-10181-3

Notice

Knowledge and best practice in this field are constantly changing. As new research and experience broaden our understanding, changes in research methods, professional practices, or medical treatment may become necessary.

Practitioners and researchers must always rely on their own experience and knowledge in evaluating and using any information, methods, compounds, or experiments described herein. In using such information or methods they should be mindful of their own safety and the safety of others, including parties for whom they have a professional responsibility.

With respect to any drug or pharmaceutical products identified, readers are advised to check the most current information provided (i) on procedures featured or (ii) by the manufacturer of each product to be administered, to verify the recommended dose or formula, the method and duration of administration, and contraindications. It is the responsibility of practitioners, relying on their own experience and knowledge of their patients, to make diagnoses, to determine dosages and the best treatment for each individual patient, and to take all appropriate safety precautions.

To the fullest extent of the law, neither the Publisher nor the authors, contributors, or editors, assume any liability for any injury and/or damage to persons or property as a matter of products liability, negligence or otherwise, or from any use or operation of any methods, products, instructions, or ideas contained in the material herein.

ISBN: 978-0-323-10181-3

Vice President, eSolutions—Nursing: *Tom Wilhelm*
Director, Simulation Solutions: *Jeff Downing*
Associate Content Development Specialist: *Sharifa Barakat*
Publishing Services Manager: *Jeffrey Patterson*
Senior Project Manager: *Tracey Schriefer*

Printed in the United States of America

Last digit is the print number: 9 8 7 6 5 4 3 2 1

Workbook
prepared by

Kelly Ann Crum, MSN, RN
Associate Faculty
Curriculum Development/Maternal Child Nursing Specialty
Health Sciences and Nursing Department
University of Phoenix, Online
Phoenix, Arizona

Textbook

Emily Slone McKinney, MSN, RN, C
Nurse Educator and Consultant
Dallas, Texas

Susan Rowen James, PhD, MSN, RN
Professor of Nursing
Curry College
Milton, Massachusetts

Sharon Smith Murray, MSN, RN
Professor Emerita, Health Professions
Golden West College
Huntington Beach, California

Kristine Ann Nelson, RN
Assistant Professor of Nursing
Tarrant County College
Trinity River East Campus Center for Health Care Professions
Fort Worth, Texas

Jean Weiler Ashwill, MSN, RN
Assistant Dean
College of Nursing
University of Texas at Arlington
Arlington, Texas

Contents

Table of Contents
McKinney, James, Murray, Nelson, and Ashwill: Maternal-Child Nursing, Fourth Edition

Pediatric Nursing Care

Getting Started

GETTING SET UP

MINIMUM SYSTEM REQUIREMENTS

WINDOWS®

Windows Vista®, XP, 2000 (Recommend Windows XP/2000)
Pentium® III processor (or equivalent) @ 600 MHz (Recommend 800 MHz or better)
256 MB of RAM (Recommend 1 GB or more for Windows Vista)
800 x 600 screen size (Recommend 1024 x 768)
Thousands of colors
12x CD-ROM drive

Note: Windows Vista and XP require administrator privileges for installation.

MACINTOSH® (Note: This CD will not work in Mac Lion 10.7)

MAC OS X (up to 10.6)
Apple Power PC G3 @ 500 MHz or better
128 MB of RAM (Recommend 256 MB or more)
800 x 600 screen size (Recommend 1024 x 768)
Thousands of colors
12x CD-ROM drive
Stereo speakers or headphones

INSTALLATION INSTRUCTIONS

WINDOWS

1. Insert the *Virtual Clinical Excursions—Obstetrics-Pediatrics* CD-ROM.
2. The setup screen should appear automatically if the current product is not already installed. Windows Vista users may be asked to authorize additional security prompts.
3. Follow the onscreen instructions during the setup process.

   If the setup screen does *not* appear automatically (and *Virtual Clinical Excursions—Obstetrics-Pediatrics* has not been installed already):
   a. Click the **My Computer** icon on your desktop or on your Start menu.
   b. Double-click on your CD-ROM drive.
   c. If installation does not start at this point:
      (1) Click the **Start** icon on the taskbar and select the **Run** option.
      (2) Type d:\setup.exe (where "d:\" is your CD-ROM drive) and press **OK**.
      (3) Follow the onscreen instructions for installation.

MACINTOSH

1. Insert the *Virtual Clinical Excursions—Obstetrics-Pediatrics* CD in the CD-ROM drive.
   The disk icon will appear on your desktop.
2. Double-click on the disk icon.
3. Double-click on the VCEOBPE_MAC run file.

Note: Virtual Clinical Excursions—Obstetrics-Pediatrics for Macintosh does not have an installation setup and can only be run directly from the CD.

HOW TO USE VIRTUAL CLINICAL EXCURSIONS—OBSTETRICS-PEDIATRICS

WINDOWS

1. Double-click on the *Virtual Clinical Excursions—Obstetrics-Pediatrics* icon located on your desktop.
2. Or navigate to the program via the Windows Start menu.

Note: If your computer uses Windows Vista, right-click on the desktop shortcut and choose **Properties**. In the Compatibility Mode, check the box for "Run as Administrator." Below is a screen capture to show what this looks like.

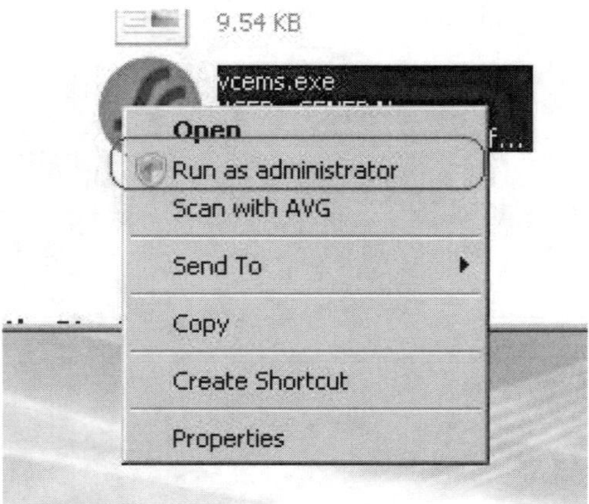

MACINTOSH

1. Insert the *Virtual Clinical Excursions—Obstetrics-Pediatrics* CD in the CD-ROM drive. The disk icon will appear on your desktop.
2. Double-click on the disk icon.
3. Double-click on the VCEOBPE_MAC run file.

SCREEN SETTINGS

For best results, your computer monitor resolution should be set at a minimum of 800 x 600. The number of colors displayed should be set to "thousands or higher" (High Color or 16 bit) or "millions of colors" (True Color or 24 bit).

Windows

1. From the **Start** menu, select **Control Panel** (on some systems, you will first go to **Settings**, then to **Control Panel**).
2. Double-click on the **Display** icon.
3. Click on the **Settings** tab.
4. Under **Screen resolution** use the slider bar to select **800 by 600 pixels**.
5. Access the **Colors** drop-down menu by clicking on the down arrow.
6. Select **High Color (16 bit)** or **True Color (24 bit)**.
7. Click on **OK**.
8. You may be asked to verify the setting changes. Click **Yes**.
9. You may be asked to restart your computer to accept the changes. Click **Yes**.

Macintosh

1. Select the **Monitors** control panel.
2. Select **800 x 600** (or similar) from the **Resolution** area.
3. Select **Thousands** or **Millions** from the **Color Depth** area.

WEB BROWSERS

Supported web browsers include Microsoft Internet Explorer (IE) version 7.0 or higher and Mozilla version 3.0 or higher.

If you use America Online® (AOL) for web access, you will need AOL version 4.0 or higher and one of the browsers listed above. Do not use earlier versions of AOL with earlier versions of IE, because you will have difficulty accessing many features.

For best results with AOL:

- Connect to the Internet using AOL version 4.0 or higher.
- Open a private chat within AOL (this allows the AOL client to remain open, without asking whether you wish to disconnect while minimized).
- Minimize AOL.
- Launch a recommended browser.

TECHNICAL SUPPORT

Technical support for this product is available 24 hours a day, seven days a week, excluding holidays. Before calling, be sure that your computer meets the minimum system requirements to run this software. Inside the United States and Canada, call 1-800-222-9570. Outside North America, call 314-447-8094. You may also fax your questions to 314-447-8078 or contact Technical Support through e-mail: technical.support@elsevier.com.

Trademarks: Windows, Macintosh, Pentium, and America Online are registered trademarks.

ACCESSING *Virtual Clinical Excursions—Obstetrics-Pediatrics* FROM EVOLVE

The product you have purchased is part of the Evolve family of online courses and learning resources. Please read the following information thoroughly to get started.

To access your instructor's course on Evolve:

Your instructor will provide you with the username and password needed to access this specific course on the Evolve Learning System. Once you have received this information, please follow these instructions:

1. Go to the Evolve student page (http://evolve.elsevier.com/student).
2. Enter your username and password in the **Login to My Evolve** area and click the **Login** button.
3. You will be taken to your personalized **My Evolve** page, where the course will be listed in the **My Courses** module.

TECHNICAL REQUIREMENTS

To use an Evolve course, you will need access to a computer that is connected to the Internet and equipped with web browser software that supports frames. For optimal performance, it is recommended that you have speakers and use a high-speed Internet connection. However, slower dial-up modems (56 K minimum) are acceptable.

Whichever browser you use, the browser preferences must be set to enable cookies and the cache must be set to reload every time.

Enable Cookies

Browser	Steps
Internet Explorer (IE) 7.0 or higher	1. Select **Tools → Internet Options**. 2. Select **Privacy** tab. 3. Use the slider (slide down) to **Accept All Cookies**. 4. Click **OK**. -OR- 3. Click the **Advanced** button. 4. Click the check box next to **Override Automatic Cookie Handling**. 5. Click the **Accept** radio buttons under **First-party Cookies** and **Third-party Cookies**. 6. Click **OK**.
Mozilla Firefox 3.0 or higher	1. Select **Tools → Options**. 2. Select the **Privacy** icon. 3. Click to expand Cookies. 4. Select **Allow sites to set cookies**. 5. Click **OK**.

Set Cache to Always Reload a Page

Browser	Steps
Internet Explorer (IE) 7.0 or higher	1. Select **Tools → Internet Options**. 2. Select **General** tab. 3. Go to the **Temporary Internet Files** and click the **Settings** button. 4. Select the radio button for **Every visit to the page** and click **OK** when complete.
Mozilla Firefox 3.0 or higher	1. Select **Tools → Options**. 2. Select the **Privacy** icon. 3. Click to expand Cache. 4. Set the value to "**0**" in the **Use up to: __ MB of disk space for the cache** field. 5. Click **OK**.

Plug-Ins

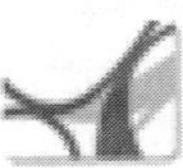

Adobe Acrobat Reader—With the free Acrobat Reader software, you can view and print Adobe PDF files. Many Evolve products offer student and instructor manuals, checklists, and more in this format!

Download at: http://www.adobe.com

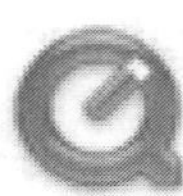

Apple QuickTime—Install this to hear word pronunciations, heart and lung sounds, and many other helpful audio clips within Evolve Online Courses!

Download at: http://www.apple.com

Adobe Flash Player—This player will enhance your viewing of many Evolve web pages, as well as educational short-form to long-form animation within the Evolve Learning System!

Download at: http://www.adobe.com

Adobe Shockwave Player—Shockwave is best for viewing the many interactive learning activities within Evolve Online Courses!

Download at: http://www.adobe.com

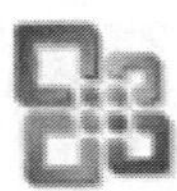

Microsoft Word Viewer—With this viewer, Microsoft Word users can share documents with those who don't have Word, and users without Word can open and view Word documents. Many Evolve products have testbank, student and instructor manuals, and other documents available for downloading and viewing on your own computer!

Download at: http://www.microsoft.com

Microsoft PowerPoint Viewer—With this viewer, you can access PowerPoint 97, 2000, and 2002 presentations even if you don't have PowerPoint. Many Evolve products have slides available for downloading and viewing on your own computer!

Download at: http://www.microsoft.com

SUPPORT INFORMATION

Live phone support is available to customers in the United States and Canada at **800-222-9570** 24 hours a day, seven days a week, excluding holidays. Support is also available through email at technical.support@elsevier.com.

Online 24/7 support can be accessed on the Evolve website (http://evolve.elsevier.com). Resources include:

- Guided tours
- Tutorials
- Frequently asked questions (FAQs)
- Online copies of course user guides
- And much more!

A QUICK TOUR

Welcome to *Virtual Clinical Excursions—Obstetrics-Pediatrics*, a virtual hospital setting in which you can work with multiple complex patient simulations and also learn to access and evaluate the information resources that are essential for high-quality patient care. The virtual hospital, Pacific View Regional Hospital, has realistic architecture and access to patient rooms, a Nurses' Station, and a Medication Room.

BEFORE YOU START

Make sure you have your textbook nearby when you use the *Virtual Clinical Excursions—Obstetrics-Pediatrics* CD. You will want to consult topic areas in your textbook frequently while working with the CD and using this workbook.

HOW TO SIGN IN

- Enter your name on the Student Nurse identification badge.
- Next, click the down arrow next to **Select Floor**. For this quick tour, choose **Obstetrics**.
- Now click the down arrow next to **Select Period of Care**. This drop-down menu gives you four periods of care from which to choose. In Periods of Care 1 through 3, you can actively engage in patient assessment, entry of data in the electronic patient record (EPR), and medication administration. Period of Care 4 presents the day in review. Highlight and click the appropriate period of care. (For this quick tour, choose **Period of Care 1: 0730-0815**.)
- Click **Go**. This takes you to the Patient List screen (see example on page 11). Note that the virtual time is provided in the box at the lower left corner of the screen (0730, since we chose Period of Care 1).

Note: If you choose to work during Period of Care 4: 1900-2000, the Patient List screen is skipped since you are not able to visit patients or administer medications during the shift. Instead, you are taken directly to the Nurses' Station, where the records of all the patients on the floor are available for your review.

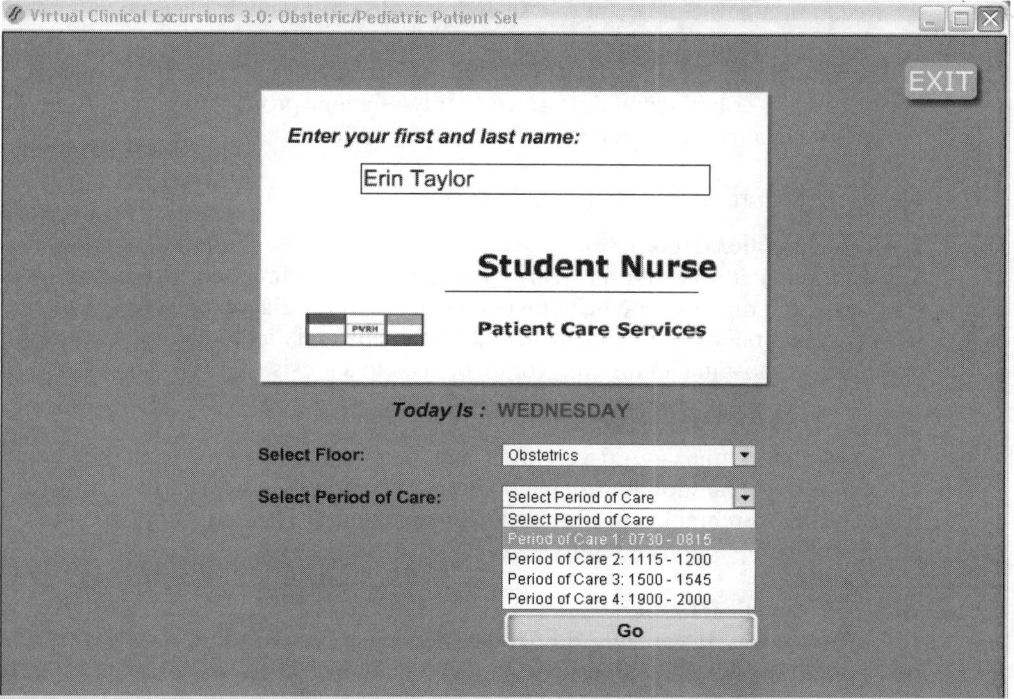

PATIENT LIST

OBSTETRICS UNIT

Dorothy Grant (Room 201)
30-week intrauterine pregnancy—A 25-year-old multipara Caucasian female admitted with abdominal trauma following a domestic violence incident. Her complications include preterm labor and extensive social issues such as acquiring safe housing for her family upon discharge.

Stacey Crider (Room 202)
27-week intrauterine pregnancy—A 21-year-old primigravida Native American female admitted for intravenous tocolysis, bacterial vaginosis, and poorly controlled insulin-dependent gestational diabetes. Strained family relationships and social isolation complicate this patient's ability to comply with strict dietary requirements and prenatal care.

Kelly Brady (Room 203)
26-week intrauterine pregnancy—A 35-year-old primigravida Caucasian female urgently admitted for progressive symptoms of preeclampsia. A history of inadequate coping with major life stressors leave her at risk for a recurrence of depression as she faces a diagnosis of HELLP syndrome and the delivery of a severely premature infant.

Maggie Gardner (Room 204)
22-week intrauterine pregnancy—A 41-year-old multigravida African-American female admitted for a high-risk pregnancy evaluation and rule out diagnosis of systemic lupus erythematosus. Coping with chronic pain, fatigue, and a history of multiple miscarriages contribute to an anxiety disorder and the need for social service intervention.

Gabriela Valenzuela (Room 205)
34-week intrauterine pregnancy—A 21-year-old primigravida Hispanic female with a history of mitral valve prolapse admitted for uterine cramping and vaginal bleeding suggestive of placental abruption following an unrestrained motor vehicle accident. Her needs include staff support for an unprepared-for labor and possible preterm birth.

Laura Wilson (Room 206)
37-week intrauterine pregnancy—An 18-year-old primigravida Caucasian female urgently admitted after being found unconscious at home. Her complications include HIV-positive status and chronic polysubstance abuse. Unrealistic expectations of parenthood and living with a chronic illness combined with strained family relations prompt comprehensive social and psychiatric evaluations initiated on the day of simulation.

PEDIATRICS UNIT

George Gonzalez (Room 301)
Diabetic ketoacidosis—An 11-year-old Hispanic male admitted for stabilization of blood glucose level and diabetic re-education associated with his diagnosis of type 1 diabetes mellitus. This patient's poor compliance with insulin therapy and dietary regime have resulted in frequent and repeated hospital admissions for diabetic ketoacidosis.

Tommy Douglas (Room 302)
Traumatic brain injury—A 6-year-old Caucasian male transferred from the Pediatric Intensive Care Unit in preparation for organ donation. This patient is status post ventriculostomy with negative intracerebral blood flow and requires extensive hemodynamic monitoring and support, along with compassionate family care.

Carrie Richards (Room 303)
Bronchiolitis—A 3½-month-old African-American female admitted with respiratory distress due to respiratory syncytial virus, along with dehydration and an inadequate nutritional status. Parent education and support are among her primary needs.

Stephanie Brown (Room 304)
Meningitis—A 3-year-old African-American female with a history of spastic cerebral palsy admitted for intravenous antibiotic therapy, neurologic monitoring, and support for a diagnosis of acute meningitis. Maintenance of physical and occupational programs addressing her mobility limitations complicate her acute care stay.

Tiffany Sheldon (Room 305)
Anorexia nervosa—A 14-year-old Caucasian female admitted for dehydration, electrolyte imbalance, and malnutrition following a syncope episode at home. This patient has a history of eating disorders, which have resulted in multiple hospital admissions and strained family dynamics between mother and daughter.

HOW TO SELECT A PATIENT

- You can choose one or more patients to work with from the Patient List by checking the box to the left of the patient name(s). For this quick tour, select Dorothy Grant. (In order to receive a scorecard for a patient, the patient must be selected before proceeding to the Nurses' Station.)
- Click on **Get Report** to the right of the medical records number (MRN) to view a summary of the patient's care during the 12-hour period before your arrival on the unit.
- After reviewing the report, click on **Go to Nurses' Station** in the right lower corner to begin your care. (*Note:* If you have been assigned to care for multiple patients, you can click on **Return to Patient List** to select and review the report for each additional patient before going to the Nurses' Station.)

Note: Even though the Patient List is initially skipped when you sign in to work for Period of Care 4, you can still access this screen if you wish to review the shift report for any of the patients. To do so, simply click on **Patient List** near the top left corner of the Nurses' Station (or click on the clipboard to the left of the Kardex). Then click on **Get Report** for the patient(s) whose care you are reviewing. This may be done during any period of care.

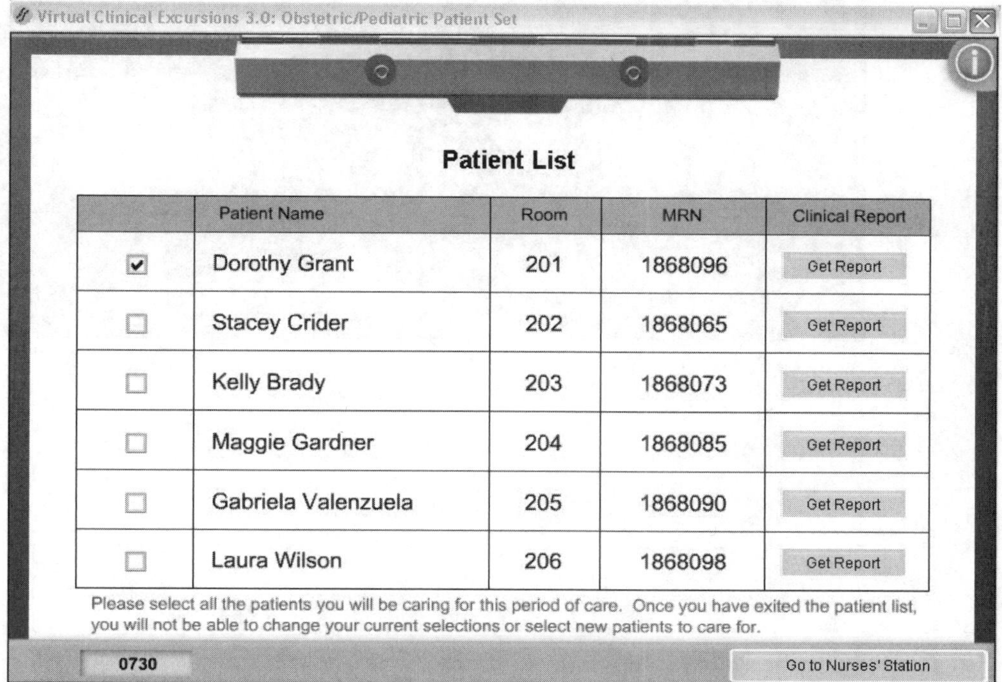

HOW TO FIND A PATIENT'S RECORDS

NURSES' STATION

Within the Nurses' Station, you will see:

1. A clipboard that contains the patient list for that floor.
2. A chart rack with patient charts labeled by room number, a notebook labeled Kardex, and a notebook labeled MAR (Medication Administration Record).
3. A desktop computer with access to the Electronic Patient Record (EPR).
4. A tool bar across the top of the screen that can also be used to access the Patient List, EPR, Chart, MAR, and Kardex. This tool bar is also accessible from each patient's room.
5. A Drug Guide containing information about the medications you are able to administer to your patients.
6. A tool bar across the bottom of the screen that can be used to access the Floor Map, patient rooms, Medication Room, and Drug Guide.

As you run your cursor over an item, it will be highlighted. To select, simply click on the item. As you use these resources, you will always be able to return to the Nurses' Station by clicking on the **Return to Nurses' Station** bar located in the right lower corner of your screen.

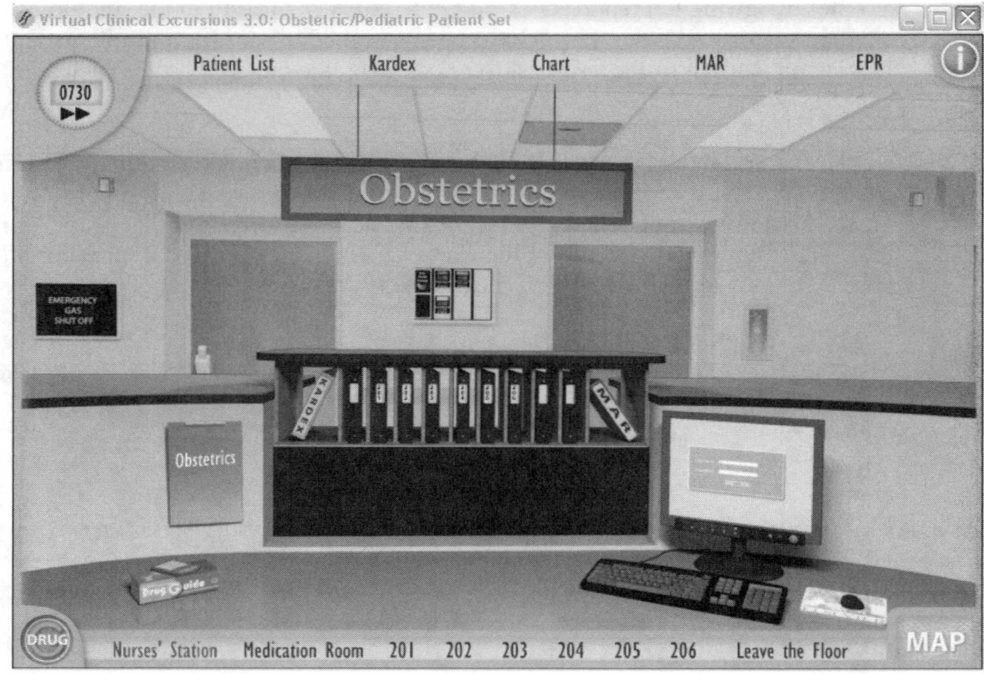

MEDICATION ADMINISTRATION RECORD (MAR)

The MAR icon located on the tool bar at the top of your screen accesses current 24-hour medications for each patient. Click on the icon and the MAR will open. (*Note:* You can also access the MAR by clicking on the MAR notebook on the far right side of the book rack in the center of the screen.) Within the MAR, tabs on the right side of the screen allow you to select patients by room number. Be careful to make sure you select the correct tab number for *your* patient rather than simply reading the first record that appears after the MAR opens. Each MAR sheet lists the following:

- Medications
- Route and dosage of each medication
- Times of administration of each medication

Note: The MAR changes each day. Expired MARs are stored in the patients' charts.

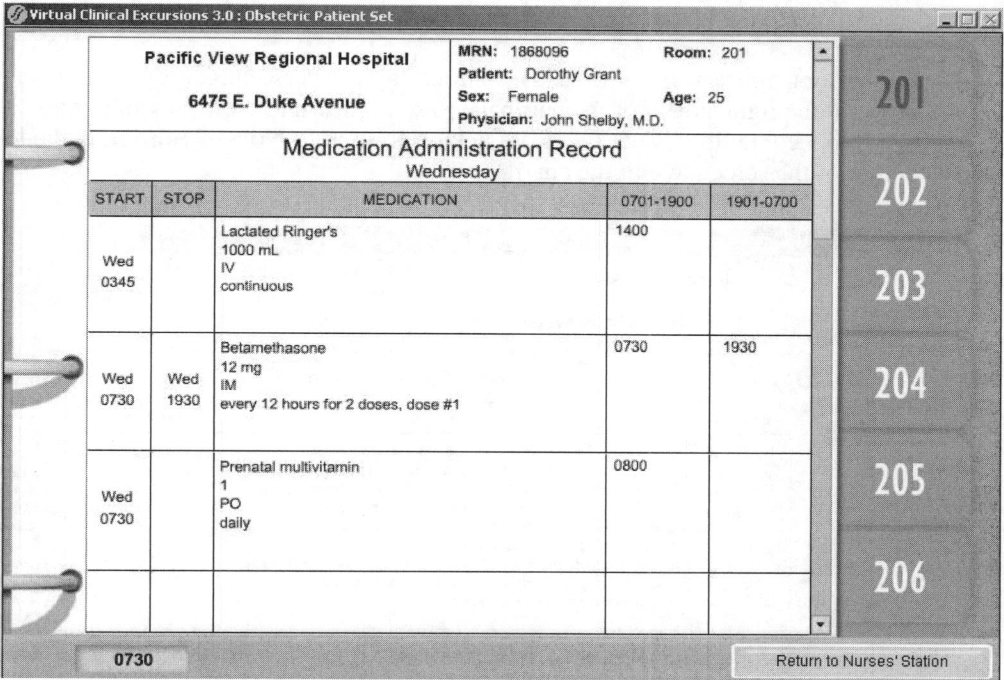

Virtual Clinical Excursions 3.0 : Obstetric Patient Set

Pacific View Regional Hospital
6475 E. Duke Avenue

MRN: 1868096 Room: 201
Patient: Dorothy Grant
Sex: Female Age: 25
Physician: John Shelby, M.D.

Medication Administration Record
Wednesday

START	STOP	MEDICATION	0701-1900	1901-0700
Wed 0345		Lactated Ringer's 1000 mL IV continuous	1400	
Wed 0730	Wed 1930	Betamethasone 12 mg IM every 12 hours for 2 doses, dose #1	0730	1930
Wed 0730		Prenatal multivitamin 1 PO daily	0800	

201 202 203 204 205 206

0730

Return to Nurses' Station

CHARTS

To access patient charts, either click on the **Chart** icon at the top of your screen or anywhere within the chart rack in the center of the Nurses' Station screen. When the close-up view appears, the individual charts are labeled by room number. To open a chart, click on the room number of the patient whose chart you wish to review. The patient's name and allergies will appear on the left side of the screen, along with a list of tabs on the right side of the screen, allowing you to view the following data:

- Allergies
- Physician's Orders
- Physician's Notes
- Nurse's Notes
- Laboratory Reports
- Diagnostic Reports
- Surgical Reports
- Consultations
- Patient Education
- History and Physical
- Nursing Admission
- Expired MARs
- Consents
- Mental Health
- Admissions
- Emergency Department

Information appears in real time. The entries are in reverse chronologic order, so use the down arrow at the right side of each chart page to scroll down to view previous entries. Flip from tab to tab to view multiple data fields or click on **Return to Nurses' Station** in the lower right corner of the screen to exit the chart.

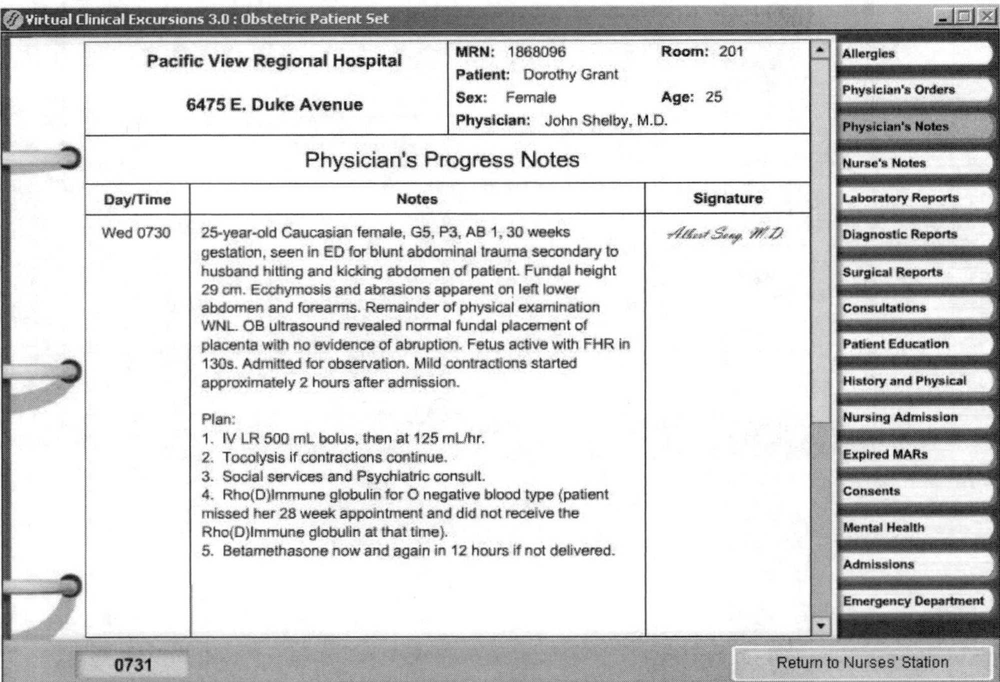

ELECTRONIC PATIENT RECORD (EPR)

The EPR can be accessed from the computer in the Nurses' Station or from the EPR icon located in the tool bar at the top of your screen. To access a patient's EPR:

- Click on either the computer screen or the **EPR** icon.
- Your username and password are automatically filled in.
- Click on **Login** to enter the EPR.
- *Note:* Like the MAR, the EPR is arranged numerically. Thus when you enter, you are initially shown the records of the patient in the lowest room number on the floor. To view the correct data for *your* patient, remember to select the correct room number, using the drop-down menu for the Patient field at the top left corner of the screen.

The EPR used in Pacific View Regional Hospital represents a composite of commercial versions being used in hospitals. You can access the EPR:

- to review existing data for a patient (by room number).
- to enter data you collect while working with a patient.

The EPR is updated daily, so no matter what day or part of a shift you are working, there will be a current EPR with the patient's data from the past days of the current hospital stay. This type of simulated EPR allows you to examine how data for different attributes have changed over time, as well as to examine data for all of a patient's attributes at a particular time. The EPR is fully functional (as it is in a real-life hospital). You can enter such data as blood pressure, breath sounds, and certain treatments. The EPR will not, however, allow you to enter data for a previous time period. Use the arrows at the bottom of the screen to move forward and backward in time.

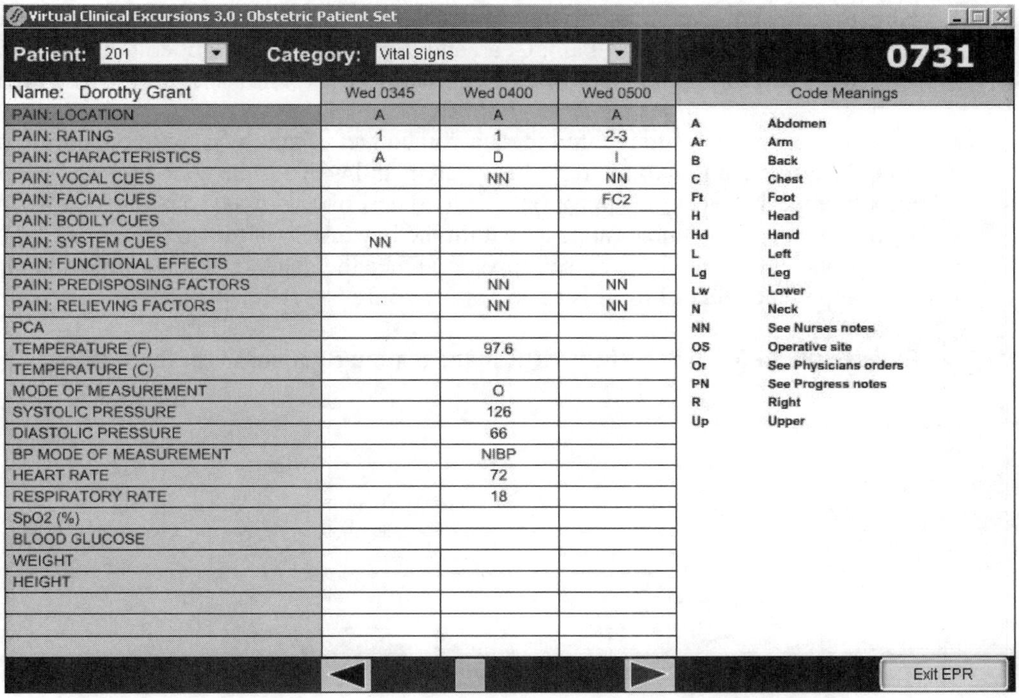

Virtual Clinical Excursions 3.0 : Obstetric Patient Set

Patient: 201 Category: Vital Signs 0731

Name: Dorothy Grant	Wed 0345	Wed 0400	Wed 0500
PAIN: LOCATION	A	A	A
PAIN: RATING	1	1	2-3
PAIN: CHARACTERISTICS	A	D	I
PAIN: VOCAL CUES		NN	NN
PAIN: FACIAL CUES			FC2
PAIN: BODILY CUES			
PAIN: SYSTEM CUES	NN		
PAIN: FUNCTIONAL EFFECTS			
PAIN: PREDISPOSING FACTORS		NN	NN
PAIN: RELIEVING FACTORS		NN	NN
PCA			
TEMPERATURE (F)		97.6	
TEMPERATURE (C)			
MODE OF MEASUREMENT		O	
SYSTOLIC PRESSURE		126	
DIASTOLIC PRESSURE		66	
BP MODE OF MEASUREMENT		NIBP	
HEART RATE		72	
RESPIRATORY RATE		18	
SpO2 (%)			
BLOOD GLUCOSE			
WEIGHT			
HEIGHT			

Code Meanings	
A	Abdomen
Ar	Arm
B	Back
C	Chest
Ft	Foot
H	Head
Hd	Hand
L	Left
Lg	Leg
Lw	Lower
N	Neck
NN	See Nurses notes
OS	Operative site
Or	See Physicians orders
PN	See Progress notes
R	Right
Up	Upper

Exit EPR

At the top of the EPR screen, you can choose patients by their room numbers. In addition, you have access to 17 different categories of patient data. To change patients or data categories, click the down arrow to the right of the room number or category.

The categories of patient data in the EPR are as follows:

- Vital Signs
- Respiratory
- Cardiovascular
- Neurologic
- Gastrointestinal
- Excretory
- Musculoskeletal
- Integumentary
- Reproductive
- Psychosocial
- Wounds and Drains
- Activity
- Hygiene and Comfort
- Safety
- Nutrition
- IV
- Intake and Output

Remember, each hospital selects its own codes. The codes used in the EPR at Pacific View Regional Hospital may be different from ones you have seen in your clinical rotations. Take some time to acquaint yourself with the codes. Within the Vital Signs category, click on any item in the left column (e.g., Pain: Characteristics). In the far-right column, you will see a list of code meanings for the possible findings and/or descriptors for that assessment area.

You will use the codes to record the data you collect as you work with patients. Click on the box in the last time column to the right of any item and wait for the code meanings applicable to that entry to appear. Select the appropriate code to describe your assessment findings and type it in the box. (*Note:* If no cursor appears within the box, click on the box again until the blue shading disappears and the blinking cursor appears.) Once the data are typed in this box, they are entered into the patient's record for this period of care only.

To leave the EPR, click on **Exit EPR** in the bottom right corner of the screen.

VISITING A PATIENT

From the Nurses' Station, click on the room number of the patient you wish to visit (in the tool bar at the bottom of your screen). Once you are inside the room, you will see a still photo of your patient in the top left corner. To verify that this is the correct patient, click on the **Check Armband** icon to the right of the photo. The patient's identification data will appear. If you click on **Check Allergies** (the next icon to the right), a list of the patient's allergies (if any) will replace the photo.

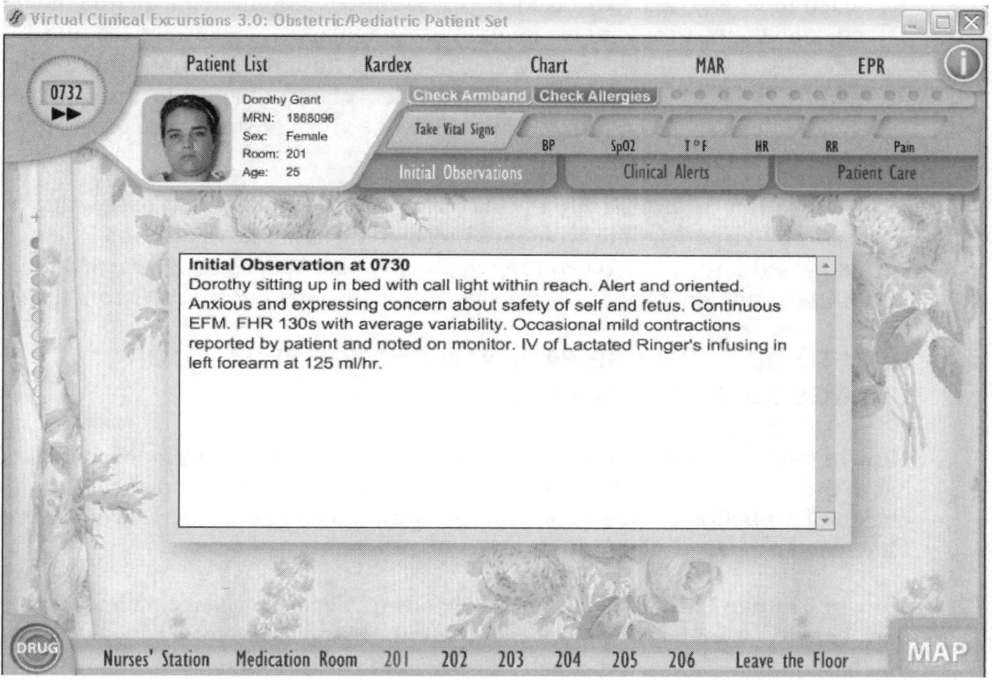

Also located in the patient's room are multiple icons you can use to assess the patient or the patient's medications. A virtual clock is provided in the upper left corner of the room to monitor your progress in real time. (*Note:* The fast-forward icon within the virtual clock will advance the time by 2-minute intervals when clicked.)

- The tool bar across the top of the screen allows you to check the **Patient List**, access the **EPR** to check or enter data, and view the patient's **Chart**, **MAR**, or **Kardex**.
- The **Take Vital Signs** icon allows you to measure the patient's up-to-the-minute blood pressure, oxygen saturation, temperature, heart rate, respiratory rate, and pain level.
- Each time you enter a patient's room, you are given an Initial Observation report to review (in the text box under the patient's photo). These notes are provided to give you a "look" at the patient as if you had just stepped into the room. You can also click on the **Initial Observations** icon to return to this box from other views within the patient's room. To the right of this icon is **Clinical Alerts**, a resource that allows you to make decisions about priority medication interventions based on emerging data collected in real time. Check this screen throughout your period of care to avoid missing critical information related to recently ordered or STAT medications.
- Clicking on **Patient Care** opens up three specific learning environments within the patient room: **Physical Assessment**, **Nurse-Client Interactions**, and **Medication Administration**.
- To perform a **Physical Assessment**, choose a body area (such as **Head & Neck**) from the column of yellow buttons. This activates a list of system subcategories for that body area (e.g., see **Sensory**, **Neurologic**, etc. in the green boxes). After you select the system you

wish to evaluate, a brief description of the assessment findings will appear in a box to the right. A still photo provides a "snapshot" of how an assessment of this area might be done or what the finding might look like. For every body area, you can also click on **Equipment** on the right side of the screen.

- To the right of the Physical Assessment icon is **Nurse-Client Interactions**. Clicking on this icon will reveal the times and titles of any videos available for viewing. (*Note:* If the video you wish to see is not listed, this means you have not yet reached the correct virtual time to view that video. Check the virtual clock; you may return to access the video once its designated time has occurred—as long as you do so within the same period of care. Or you can click on the fast-forward icon within the virtual clock to advance the time by 2-minute intervals. You will then need to click again on **Patient Care** and **Nurse-Client Interactions** to refresh the screen.) To view a listed video, click on the white arrow to the right of the video title. Use the control buttons below the video to start, stop, pause, rewind, or fast-forward the action or to mute the sound.
- **Medication Administration** is the pathway that allows you to review and administer medications to a patient after you have prepared them in the Medication Room. This process is addressed further in *How to Prepare Medications* (pages 19-20), in *Medications* (pages 26-30) For additional hands-on practice, see *Reducing Medication Errors* (pages 37-41).

HOW TO QUIT, CHANGE PATIENTS, CHANGE FLOORS, OR CHANGE PERIODS OF CARE

How to Quit: From most screens, you may click the **Leave the Floor** icon on the bottom tool bar to the right of the patient room numbers. (*Note:* From some screens, you will first need to click an **Exit** button or **Return to Nurses' Station** before clicking **Leave the Floor**.) When the Floor Menu appears, click **Exit** to leave the program.

How to Change Patients, Floors, or Periods of Care: To change patients, simply click on the new patient's room number. (You cannot receive a scorecard for a new patient, however, unless you have already selected that patient on the Patient List screen.) To change to a new period of care, to change floors, or to restart the virtual clock, click on **Leave the Floor** and then on **Restart the Program**.

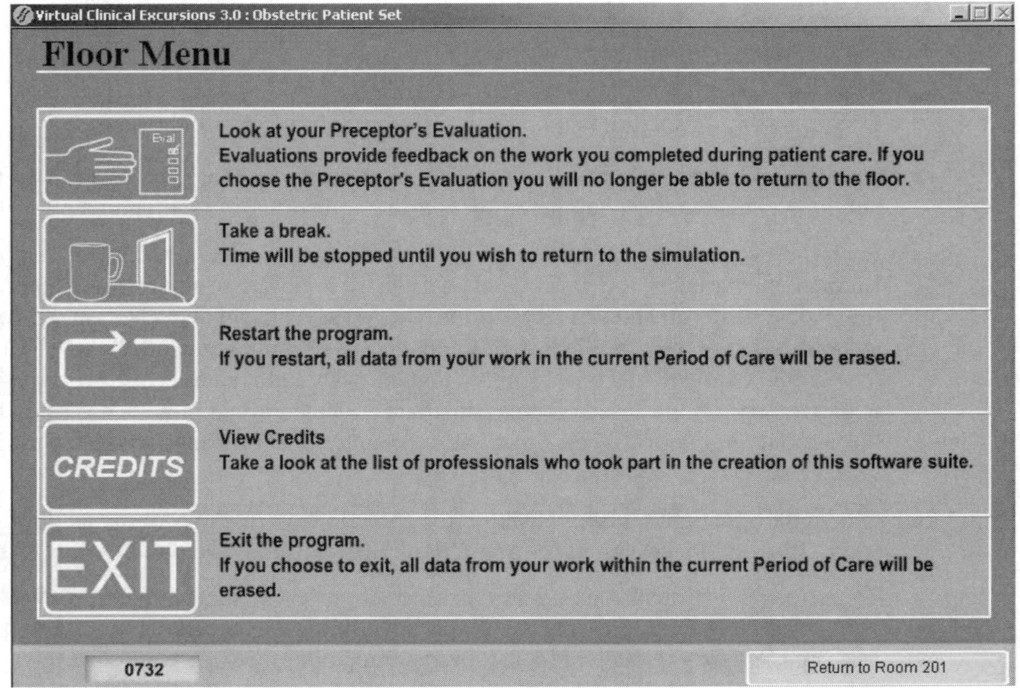

HOW TO PREPARE MEDICATIONS

From the Nurses' Station or the patient's room, you can access the Medication Room by clicking on the icon in the tool bar at the bottom of your screen to the left of the patient room numbers.

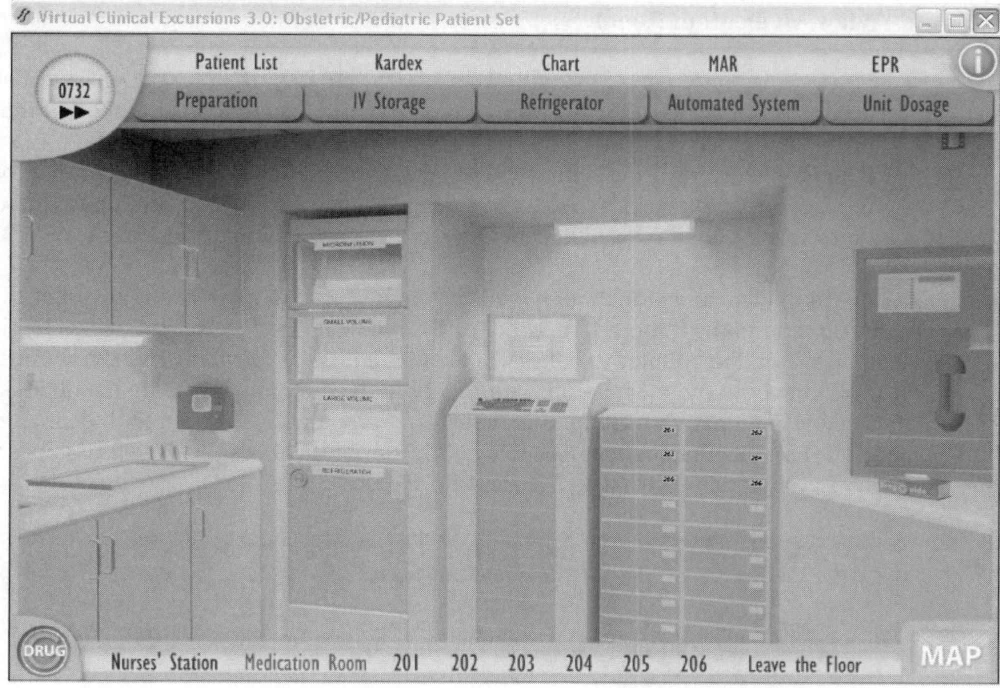

In the Medication Room you have access to the following (from left to right):

- A preparation area is located on the counter under the cabinets. To begin the medication preparation process, click on the tray on the counter or click on the **Preparation** icon at the top of the screen. The next screen leads you through a specific sequence (called the Preparation Wizard) to prepare medications one at a time for administration to a patient. However, no medication has been selected at this time. We will do this while working with a patient in *A Detailed Tour*. To exit this screen, click on **View Medication Room**.

- To the right of the cabinets (and above the refrigerator), IV storage bins are provided. Click on the bins themselves or on the **IV Storage** icon at the top of the screen. The bins are labeled **Microinfusion**, **Small Volume**, and **Large Volume**. Click on an individual bin to see a list of its contents. If you needed to prepare an IV medication at this time, you could click on the medication and its label would appear to the right under the patient's name. (*Note:* You can **Open** and **Close** any medication label by clicking the appropriate icon.) Next, you would click **Put Medication on Tray**. If you ever change your mind or decide that you have put the incorrect medication on the tray, you can reverse your actions by highlighting the medication on the tray and then clicking **Put Medication in Bin**. Click **Close Bin** in the right bottom corner to exit. **View Medication Room** brings you back to a full view of the entire room.

- A refrigerator is located under the IV storage bins to hold any medications that must be stored below room temperature. Click on the refrigerator door or on the **Refrigerator** icon at the top of the screen. Then click on the close-up view of the door to access the medications. When you are finished, click **Close Door** and then **View Medication Room**.

- To prepare controlled substances, click the **Automated System** icon at the top of the screen or click the computer monitor located to the right of the IV storage bins. A login screen will appear; your name and password are automatically filled in. Click **Login**. Select the patient for whom you wish to access medications; then select the correct medication drawer to open (they are stored alphabetically). Click **Open Drawer**, highlight the proper medication, and choose **Put Medication on Tray**. When you are finished, click **Close Drawer** and then **View Medication Room**.

- Next to the Automated System is a set of drawers identified by patient room number. To access these, click on the drawers or on the **Unit Dosage** icon at the top of the screen. This provides a close-up view of the drawers. To open a drawer, click on the room number of the patient you are working with. Next, click on the medication you would like to prepare for the patient, and a label will appear, listing the medication strength, units, and dosage per unit. To exit, click **Close Drawer**; then click **View Medication Room**.

At any time, you can learn about a medication you wish to prepare for a patient by clicking on the **Drug** icon in the bottom left corner of the medication room screen or by clicking the **Drug Guide** book on the counter to the right of the unit dosage drawers. The **Drug Guide** provides information about the medications commonly included in nursing drug handbooks. Nutritional supplements and maintenance intravenous fluid preparations are not included. Highlight a medication in the alphabetical list; relevant information about the drug will appear in the screen below. To exit, click **Return to Medication Room**.

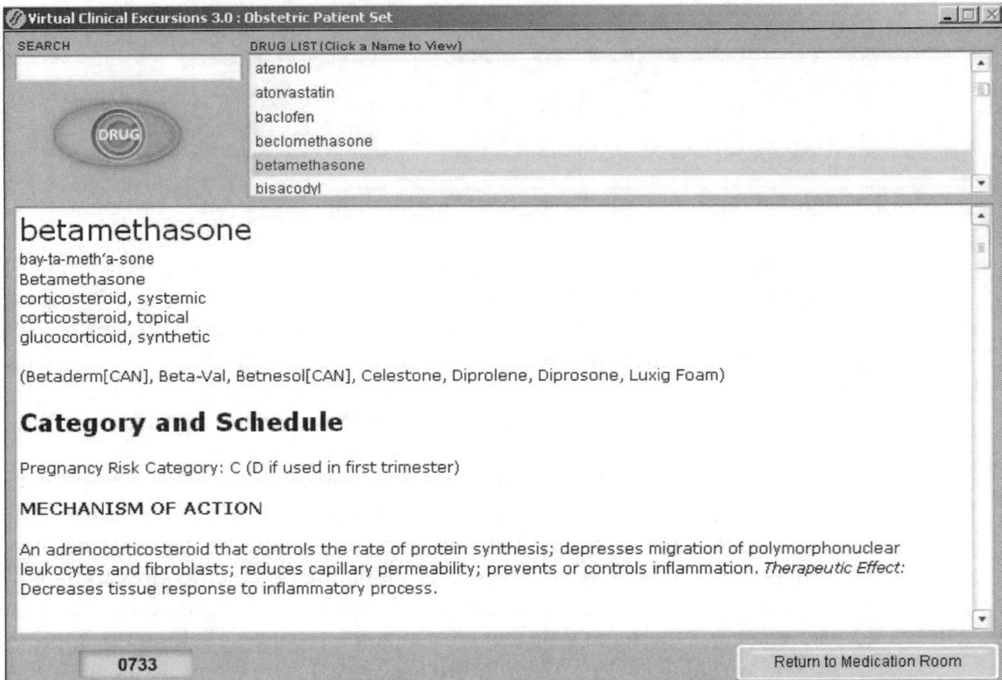

To access the MAR from the Medication Room and to review the medications ordered for a patient, click on the **MAR** icon located in the tool bar at the top of your screen and then click on the correct tab for your patient's room number. You may also click the **Review MAR** icon in the tool bar at the bottom of your screen from inside each medication storage area.

After you have chosen and prepared medications, go to the patient's room to administer them by clicking on the room number in the bottom tool bar. Inside the patient's room, click **Patient Care** and then **Medication Administration** and follow the proper administration sequence.

PRECEPTOR'S EVALUATIONS

When you have finished a session, click on **Leave the Floor** to go to the Floor Menu. At this point, you can click on the top icon (**Look at Your Preceptor's Evaluation**) to receive a scorecard that provides feedback on the work you completed during patient care.

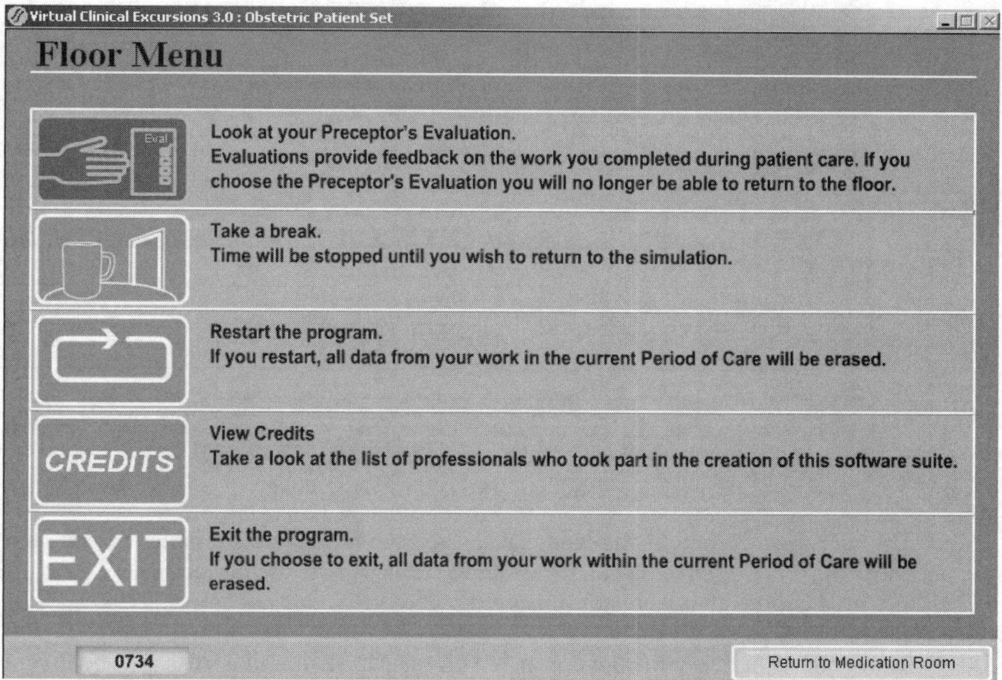

Evaluations are available for each patient you selected when you signed in for the current period of care. Click on the **Medication Scorecard** icon to see an example.

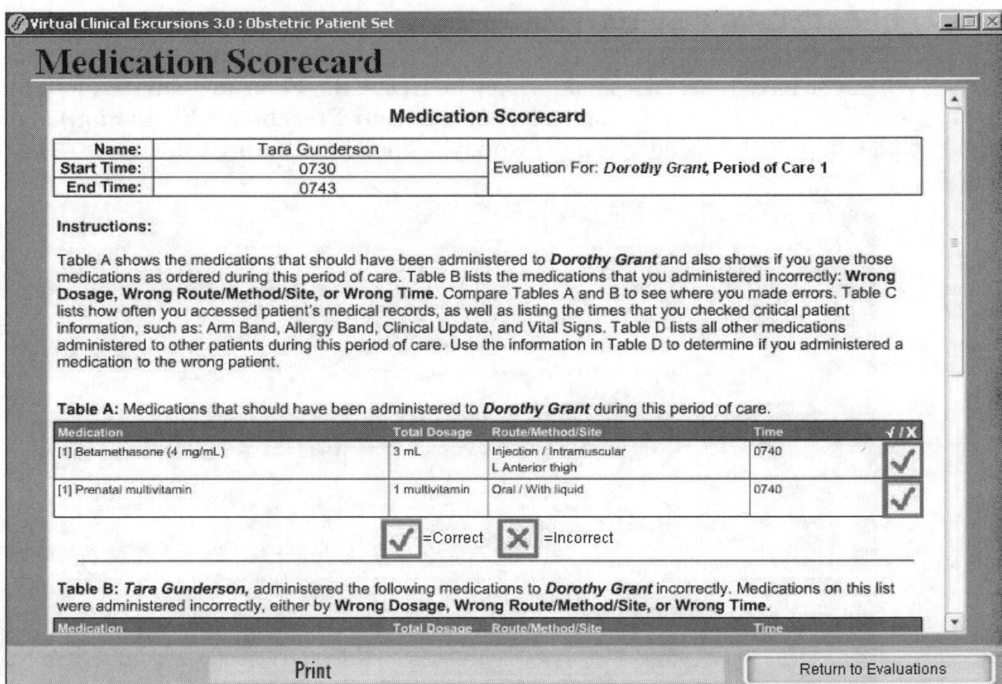

The scorecard compares the medications you administered to a patient during a period of care with what should have been administered. Table A lists the correct medications. Table B lists any medications that were administered incorrectly.

Remember, not every medication listed on the MAR should necessarily be given. For example, a patient might have an allergy to a drug that was ordered, or a medication might have been improperly transcribed to the MAR. Predetermined medication "errors" embedded within the program challenge you to exercise critical thinking skills and professional judgment when deciding to administer a medication, just as you would in a real hospital. Use all your available resources, such as the patient's chart and the MAR, to make your decision.

Table C lists the resources that were available to assist you in medication administration. It also documents whether and when you accessed these resources. For example, did you check the patient armband or perform a check of vital signs? If so, when?

You can click **Print** to get a copy of this report if needed. When you have finished reviewing the scorecard, click **Return to Evaluations** and then **Return to Menu**.

FLOOR MAP

To get a general sense of your location within the hospital, you can click on the **Map** icon found in the lower right corner of most of the screens in the *Virtual Clinical Excursions—Obstetrics-Pediatrics* program. (*Note:* If you are following this quick tour step by step, you will need to **Restart the Program** from the Floor Menu, sign in again, and go to the Nurses' Station to access the map.) When you click the **Map** icon, a floor map appears, showing the layout of the floor you are currently on, as well as a directory of the patients and services on that floor. As you move your cursor over the directory list, the location of each room is highlighted on the map (and vice versa). The floor map can be accessed from the Nurses' Station, Medication Room, and each patient's room.

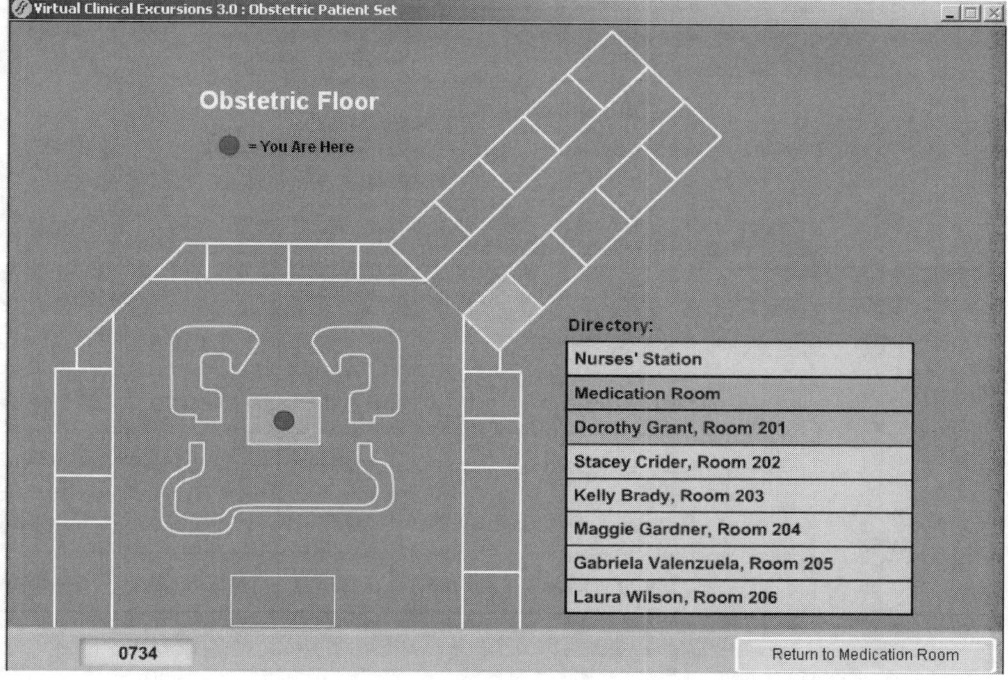

A DETAILED TOUR

If you wish to more thoroughly understand the capabilities of *Virtual Clinical Excursions—Obstetrics-Pediatrics*, take a detailed tour by completing the following section. During this tour, we will work with a specific patient to introduce you to all the different components and learning opportunities available within the software.

■ WORKING WITH A PATIENT

Sign in to work on the Obstetrics Floor for Period of Care 1 (0730-0815). From the Patient List, select Dorothy Grant in Room 201; however, do not go to the Nurses' Station yet.

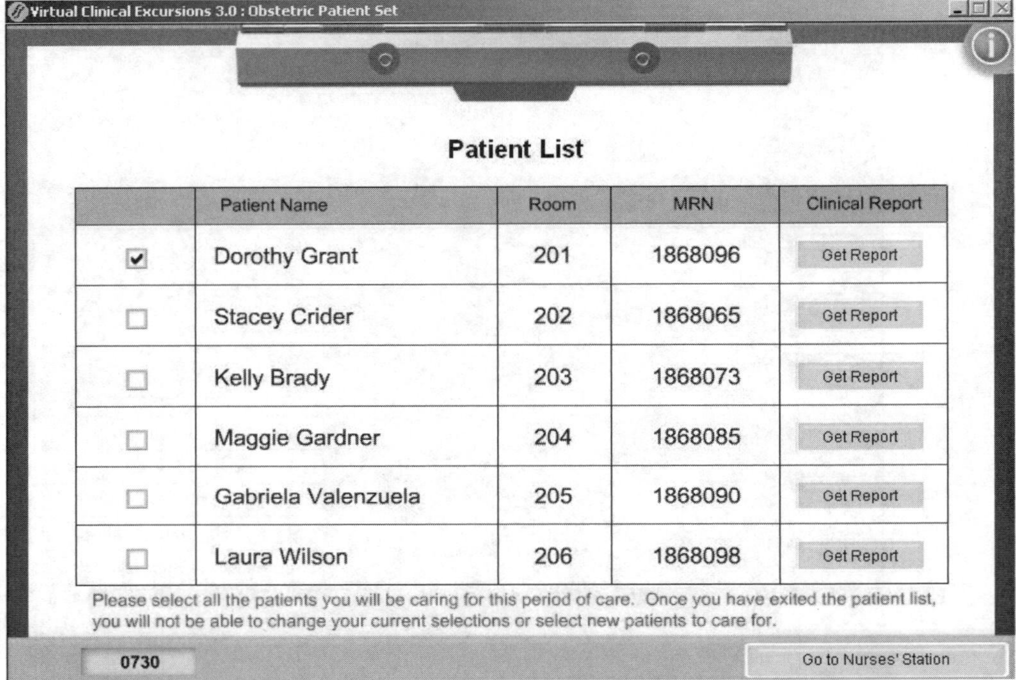

■ REPORT

In hospitals, when one shift ends and another begins, the outgoing nurse who attended a patient will give a verbal and sometimes a written summary of that patient's condition to the incoming nurse who will assume care for the patient. This summary is called a report and is an important source of data to provide an overview of a patient. Your first task is to get the clinical report on Dorothy Grant. To do this, click **Get Report** in the far right column in this patient's row. From a brief review of this summary, identify the problems and areas of concern that you will need to address for this patient.

When you have finished noting any areas of concern, click **Go to Nurses' Station**.

CHARTS

You can access Dorothy Grant's chart from the Nurses' Station or from the patient's room (201). From the Nurses' Station, click on the chart rack or on the **Chart** icon in the tool bar at the top of your screen. Next, click on the chart labeled **201** to open the medical record for Dorothy Grant. Click on the **Emergency Department** tab to view a record of why this patient was admitted.

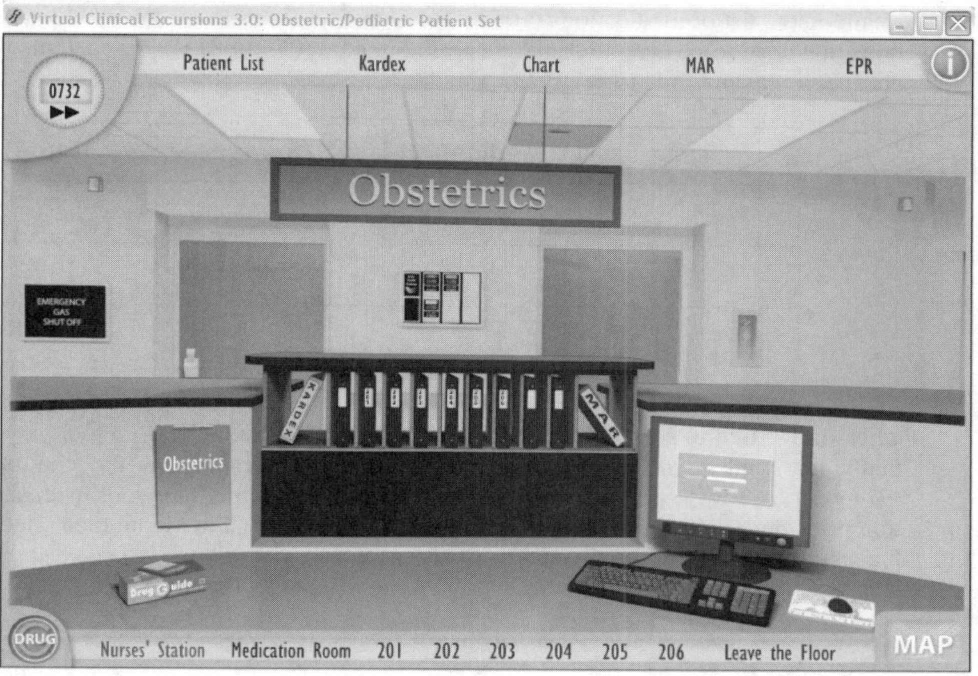

How many days has Dorothy Grant been in the hospital?

What tests were done upon her arrival in the Emergency Department and why?

What was the reason for her admission?

You should also click on **Diagnostic Reports** to learn what additional tests or procedures were performed and when. Finally, review the **Nursing Admission** and **History and Physical** to learn about the health history of this patient. When you are done reviewing the chart, click **Return to Nurses' Station**.

MEDICATIONS

Open the Medication Administration Record (MAR) by clicking on the **MAR** icon in the tool bar at the top of your screen. *Remember:* The MAR automatically opens to the first occupied room number on the floor—which is not necessarily your patient's room number! Since you need to access Dorothy Grant's MAR, click on tab **201** (her room number). Always make sure you are giving the *Right Drug to the Right Patient!*

Examine the list of medications ordered for Dorothy Grant. In the table below, list the medications that need to be given during this period of care (0730-0815). For each medication, note the dosage, route, and time to be given.

Time	Medication	Dosage	Route

Click on **Return to Nurses' Station**. Next, click on **201** on the bottom tool bar and then verify that you are indeed in Dorothy Grant's room. Select **Clinical Alerts** (the icon to the right of Initial Observations) to check for any emerging data that might affect your medication administration priorities. Next, go to the patient's chart (click on the **Chart** icon; then click on **201**). When the chart opens, select the **Physician's Orders** tab.

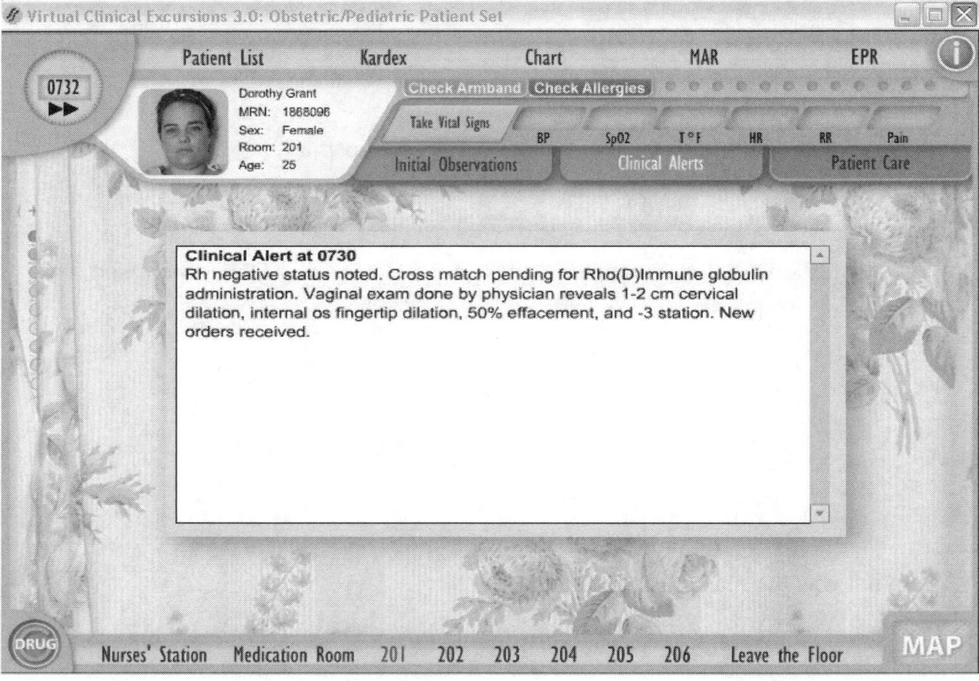

Review the orders. Have any new medications been ordered? Return to the MAR (click **Return to Room 201**; then click **MAR**). Verify that any new medications have been correctly transcribed to the MAR. Mistakes are sometimes made in the transcription process in the hospital setting, and it is sound practice to double-check any new order.

Are there any patient assessments you will need to perform before administering these medications? If so, return to Room 201 and click on **Patient Care** and then **Physical Assessment** to complete those assessments before proceeding.

Now click on the **Medication Room** icon in the tool bar at the bottom of your screen to locate and prepare the medications for Dorothy Grant.

In the Medication Room, you must access the medications for Dorothy Grant from the specific dispensing system in which each medication is stored. Locate each medication that needs to be given in this time period and click on **Put Medication on Tray** as appropriate. (*Hint:* Look in **Unit Dosage** drawer first.) When you are finished, click on **Close Drawer** and then on **View Medication Room**. Now click on the medication tray on the counter on the left side of the medication room screen to begin preparing the medications you have selected. (*Remember:* You can also click **Preparation** in the tool bar at the top of screen.)

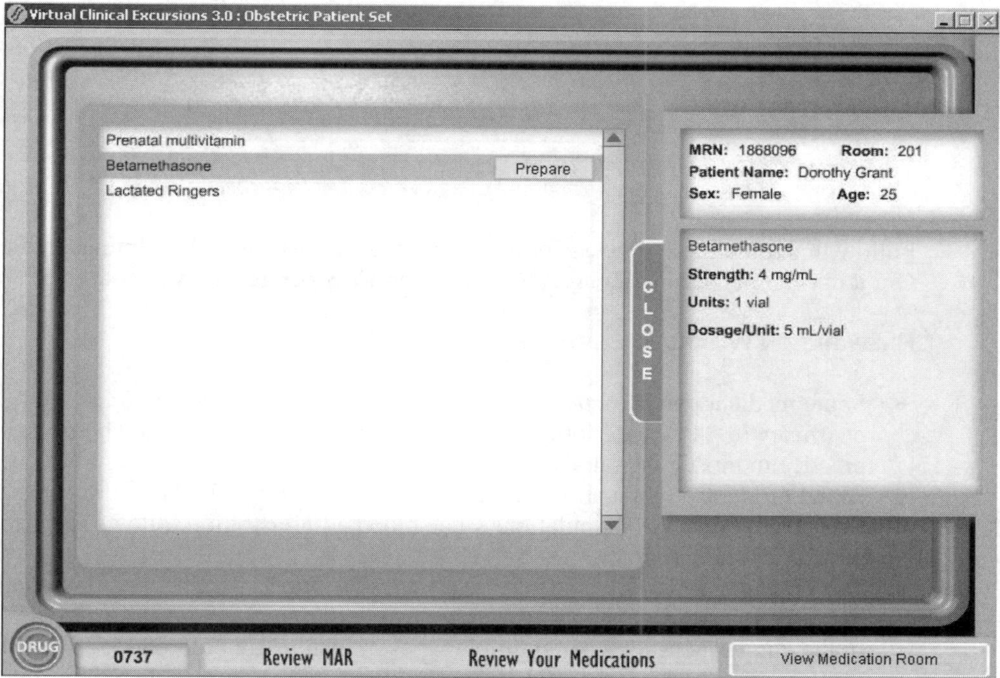

In the preparation area, you should see a list of the medications you put on the tray in the previous steps. Click on the first medication and then click **Prepare**. Follow the onscreen instructions of the Preparation Wizard, providing any data requested. As an example, let's follow the preparation process for betamethasone, one of the medications due to be administered to Dorothy Grant during this period of care. To begin, click on **Betamethasone**; then click **Prepare**. Now work through the Preparation Wizard sequence as detailed below:

Amount of medication in the ampule: 5 mL.
Enter the amount of medication you will draw up into a syringe: **3** mL.
Click **Next**.
Select the patient you wish to set aside the medication for: **Room 201, Dorothy Grant**.
Click **Finish**.
Click **Return to Medication Room**.

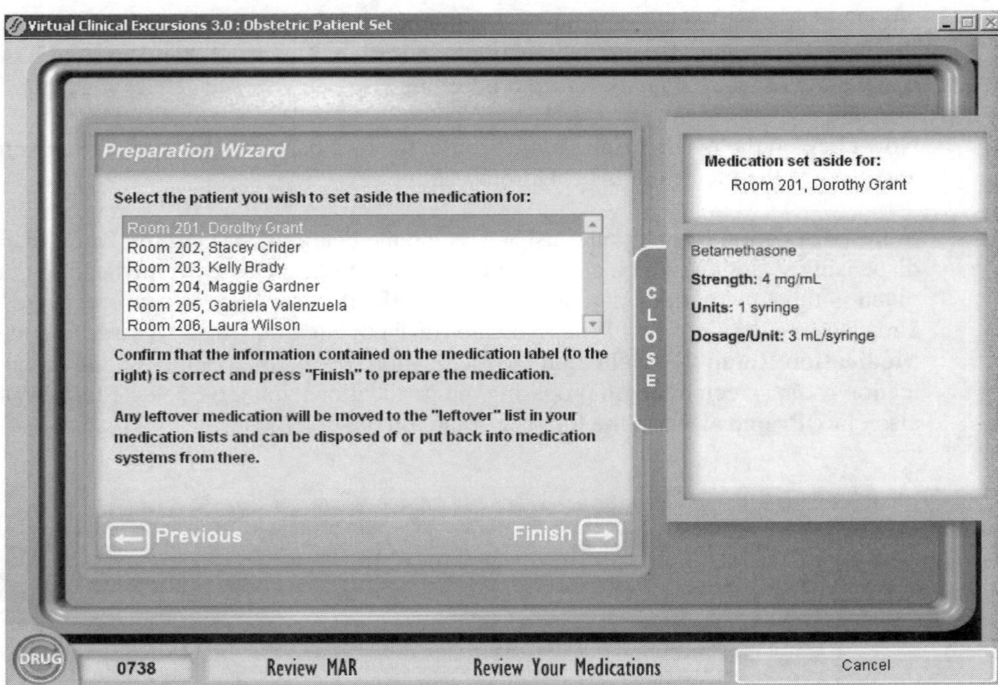

Follow this same basic process for the other medications due to be administered to Dorothy Grant during this period of care. (*Hint:* Look in **IV Storage** and **Automated System**.)

PREPARATION WIZARD EXCEPTIONS

- Some medications in *Virtual Clinical Excursions—Obstetrics-Pediatrics* are prepared by the pharmacy (e.g., IV antibiotics) and taken to the patient room as a whole. This is common practice in most hospitals.
- Blood products are not administered by students through the *Virtual Clinical Excursions—Obstetrics-Pediatrics* simulations since blood administration follows specific protocols not covered in this program.
- The *Virtual Clinical Excursions—Obstetrics-Pediatrics* simulations do not allow for mixing more than one type of medication, such as regular and Lente insulins, in the same syringe. In the clinical setting, when multiple types of insulin are ordered for a patient, the regular insulin is drawn up first, followed by the longer-acting insulin. Insulin is always administered in a special unit-marked syringe.

Now return to Room 201 (click on **201** on the bottom tool bar) to administer Dorothy Grant's medications.

At any time during the medication administration process, you can perform a further review of systems, take vital signs, check information contained within the chart, or verify patient identity and allergies. Inside Dorothy Grant's room, click **Take Vital Signs**. (*Note:* These findings change over time to reflect the temporal changes you would find in a patient similar to Dorothy Grant.)

When you have gathered all the data you need, click on **Patient Care** and then select **Medication Administration**. Any medications you prepared in the previous steps should be listed on the left side of your screen. Let's continue the administration process with the betamethasone ordered for Dorothy Grant. Click to highlight **Betamethasone** in the list of medications. Next, click on the down arrow to the right of **Select** and choose **Administer** from the drop-down menu. This will activate the Administration Wizard. Complete the Wizard sequence as follows:

- Route: **Injection**
- Method: **Intramuscular**
- Site: **Any**
- Click **Administer to Patient** arrow.
- Would you like to document this administration in the MAR? **Yes**
- Click **Finish** arrow.

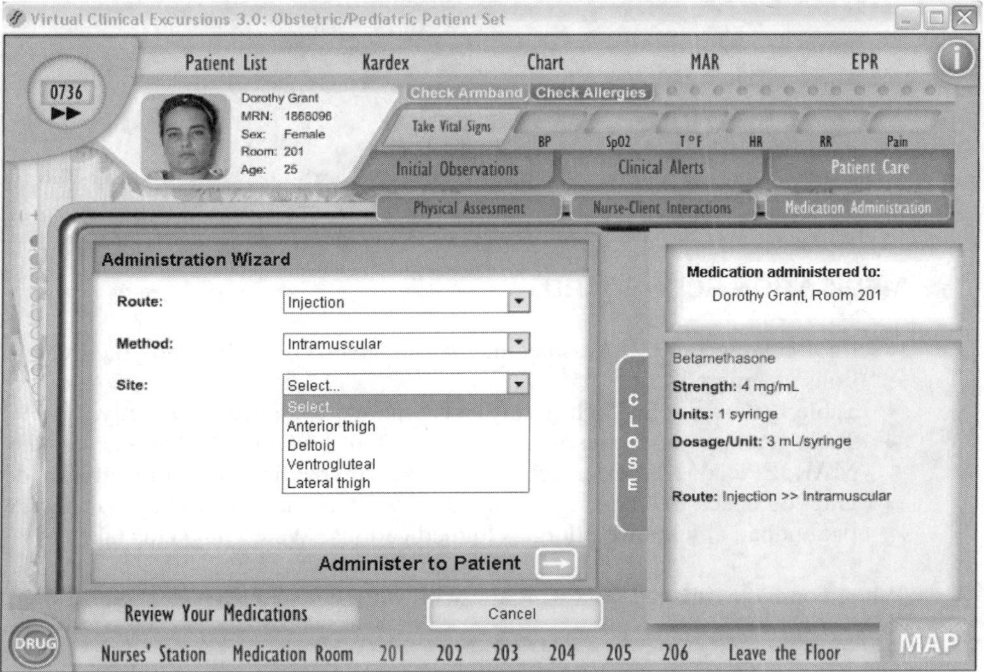

Your selections are recorded by a tracking system and evaluated on a Medication Scorecard stored under Preceptor's Evaluations. This scorecard can be viewed, printed, and given to your instructor. To access the Preceptor's Evaluations, click on **Leave the Floor**. When the Floor Menu appears, select **Look at Your Preceptor's Evaluation**. Then click on **Medication Scorecard** inside the box with Dorothy Grant's name (see example on the following page).

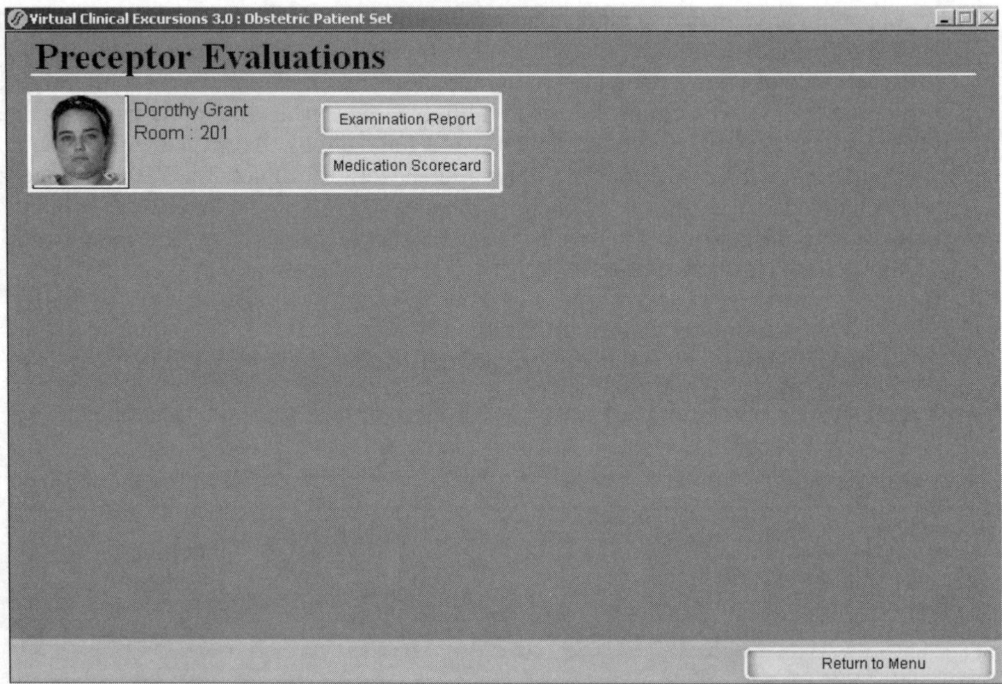

■ MEDICATION SCORECARD

- First, review Table A. Was betamethasone given correctly? Did you give the other medications as ordered?
- Table B shows you which (if any) medications you gave incorrectly.
- Table C addresses the resources used for Dorothy Grant. Did you access the patient's chart, MAR, EPR, or Kardex as needed to make safe medication administration decisions?
- Did you check the patient's armband to verify her identity? Did you check whether your patient had any known allergies to medications? Were vital signs taken?

When you have finished reviewing the scorecard, click **Return to Evaluations** and then **Return to Menu**.

■ VITAL SIGNS

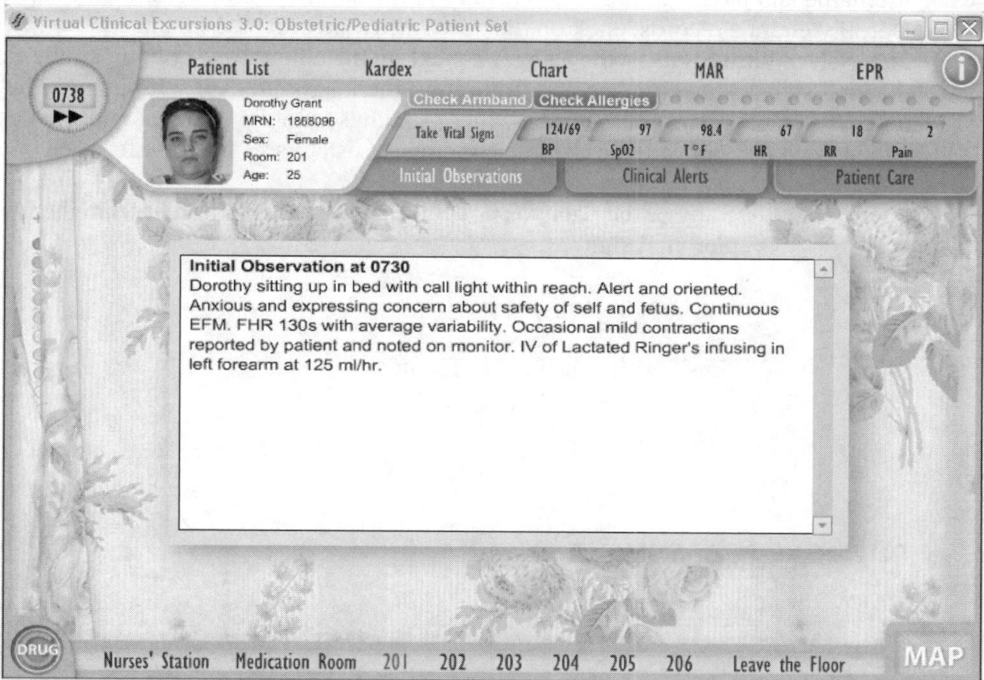

Vital signs, often considered the traditional "signs of life," include body temperature, heart rate, respiratory rate, blood pressure, oxygen saturation of the blood, and pain level.

Inside Dorothy Grant's room, click **Take Vital Signs**. (*Note:* If you are following this detailed tour step by step, you will need to **Restart the Program** from the Floor Menu, sign in again for Period of Care 1, and navigate to Room 201.) Collect vital signs for this patient and record them below. Note the time at which you collected each of these data. (*Remember:* You can take vital signs at any time. The data change over time to reflect the temporal changes you would find in a patient similar to Dorothy Grant.)

Vital Signs	Findings/Time
Blood pressure	
O_2 saturation	
Temperature	
Heart rate	
Respiratory rate	
Pain rating	

After you are done, click on the **EPR** icon located in the tool bar at the top of the screen. Your username and password are automatically provided. Click on **Login** to enter the EPR. To access Dorothy Grant's records, click on the down arrow next to Patient and choose her room number, **201**. Select **Vital Signs** as the category. Next, in the empty time column on the far right, record the vital signs data you just collected in the patient's room. (*Note:* If you need help with this process, see page 16.) Now compare these findings with the data you collected earlier for this patient's vital signs. Use these earlier findings to establish a baseline for each of the vital signs.

a. Are any of the data you collected significantly different from the baseline for a particular vital sign?

Circle One: Yes No

b. If "Yes," which data are different?

PHYSICAL ASSESSMENT

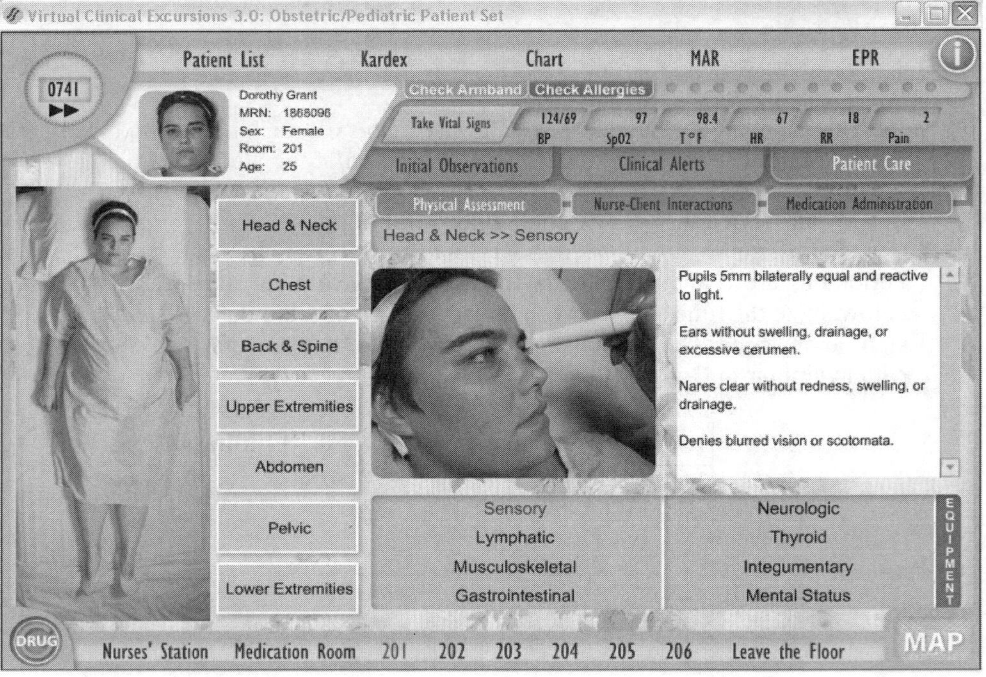

After you have finished examining the EPR for vital signs, click **Exit EPR** to return to Room 201. Click **Patient Care** and then **Physical Assessment**. Think about the information you received in the report at the beginning of this shift, as well as what you may have learned about this patient from the chart. Based on this, what area(s) of examination should you pay most attention to at this time? Is there any equipment you should be monitoring? Conduct a physical assessment of the body areas and systems that you consider priorities for Dorothy Grant. For example, select **Head & Neck**; then click on and assess **Sensory** and **Lymphatic**. Complete any other assessment(s) you think are necessary at this time. In the following table, record the data you collected during this examination.

Area of Examination	Findings
Head & Neck Sensory	
Head & Neck Lymphatic	

After you have finished collecting these data, return to the EPR. Compare the data that were already in the record with those you just collected.

a. Are any of the data you collected significantly different from the baselines for this patient?

   Circle One: Yes No

b. If "Yes," which data are different?

■ NURSE-CLIENT INTERACTIONS

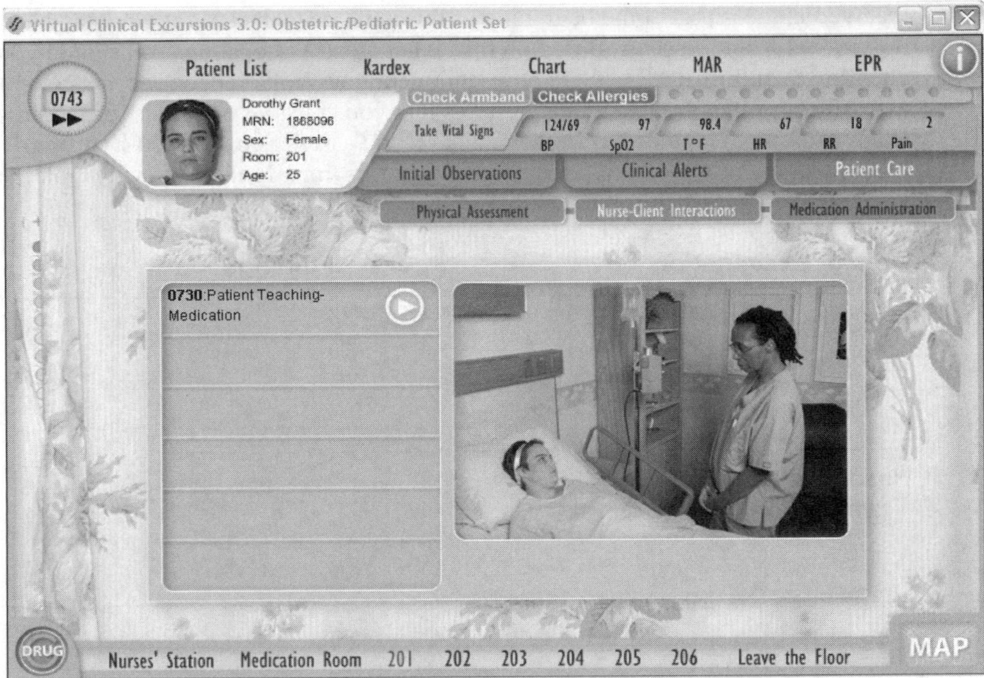

Click on **Patient Care** from inside Dorothy Grant's room (201). Now click on **Nurse-Client Interactions** to access a short video titled **Patient Teaching—Medication**, which is available for viewing at or after 0730 (based on the virtual clock in the upper left corner of your screen; see *Note* below). To begin the video, click on the white arrow next to its title. You will observe a nurse communicating with Dorothy Grant. There are many variations of nursing practice, some exemplifying "best" practice and some not. Note whether the nurse in this interaction displays professional behavior and compassionate care. Are her words congruent with what is going on with the patient? Does this interaction "feel right" to you? If not, how would you handle this situation differently? Explain.

Note: If the video you wish to view is not listed, this means you have not yet reached the correct virtual time to view that video. Check the virtual clock; you may return to access the video once its designated time has occurred—as long as you do so within the same period of care. Or you can click on the fast-forward icon within the virtual clock to advance the time by 2-minute intervals. You will then need to click again on **Patient Care** and **Nurse-Client Interactions** to refresh the screen.

At least one Nurse-Client Interactions video is available during each period of care. Viewing these videos can help you learn more about what is occurring with a patient at a certain time and also prompt you to discern between nurse communications that are ideal and those that need improvement. Compassionate care and the ability to communicate clearly are essential components of delivering quality nursing care, and it is during your clinical time that you will begin to refine these skills.

COLLECTING AND EVALUATING DATA

Each of the activities you perform in the Patient Care environment generates a significant amount of assessment data. Remember that after you collect data, you can record your findings in the EPR. You can also review the EPR, patient's chart, videos, and MAR at any time. You will get plenty of practice collecting and then evaluating data in context of the patient's course.

Now, here's an important question for you:

> Did the previous sequence of exercises provide the most efficient way to assess Dorothy Grant?

For example, you went to the patient's room to get vital signs, then back to the EPR to enter data and compare your findings with extant data. Next, you went back to the patient's room to do a physical examination, then again back to the EPR to enter and review data. If this back-and-forth process of data collection and recording seemed inefficient, remember the following:

- Plan all of your nursing activities to maximize efficiency, while at the same time optimizing the quality of patient care. (Think about what data you might need before performing certain tasks. For example, do you need to check a heart rate before administering a cardiac medication or check an IV site before starting an infusion?)
- You collect a tremendous amount of data when you work with a patient. Very few people can accurately remember all these data for more than a few minutes. Develop efficient assessment skills, and record data as soon as possible after collecting them.
- Assessment data are only the starting point for the nursing process.

Make a clear distinction between these first exercises and how you actually provide nursing care. These initial exercises were designed to involve you actively in the use of different software components. This workbook focuses on sensible practices for implementing the nursing process in ways that ensure the highest-quality care of patients.

Most important, remember that a human being changes through time, and that these changes include both the physical and psychosocial facets of a person as a living organism. Think about this for a moment. Some patients may change physically in a very short time (a patient with emerging myocardial infarction) or more slowly (a patient with a chronic illness). Patients' overall physical and psychosocial conditions may improve or deteriorate. They may have effective coping skills and familial support, or they may feel alone and full of despair. In fact, each individual is a complex mix of physical and psychosocial elements, and at least some of these elements usually change through time.

Thus it is crucial that you *DO NOT* think of the nursing process as a simple one-time, five-step procedure consisting of assessment, nursing diagnosis, planning, implementation, and evaluation. Rather, the nursing process should be utilized as a creative and systematic approach to delivering nursing care. Furthermore, because all living organisms are constantly changing, we must apply the nursing process over and over. Each time we follow the nursing process for an individual patient, we refine our understanding of that patient's physical and psychosocial conditions based on collection and analysis of many different types of data. *Virtual Clinical Excursions—Obstetrics-Pediatrics* will help you develop both the creativity and the systematic approach needed to become a nurse who is equipped to deliver the highest-quality care to all patients.

REDUCING MEDICATION ERRORS

Earlier in this detailed tour, you learned the basic steps of medication preparation and administration. The following simulations will allow you to practice those skills further—with an increased emphasis on reducing medication errors by using the Medication Scorecard to evaluate your work.

Sign in to work on the Obstetrics Floor at Pacific View Regional Hospital for Period of Care 1. (*Note:* If you are already working with another patient or during another period of care, click on **Leave the Floor** and then **Restart the Program**; then sign in.)

From the Patient List, select Dorothy Grant. Then click on **Go to Nurses' Station**. Complete the following steps to prepare and administer medications to Dorothy Grant.

- Click on **Medication Room** on the tool bar at the bottom of your screen.
- Click on **MAR** and then on tab **201** to determine medications that have been ordered for Dorothy Grant. (*Note:* You may click on **Review MAR** at any time to verify the correct medication order. Always remember to check the patient name on the MAR to make sure you have the correct patient's record. You must click on the correct room number tab within the MAR.) Click on **Return to Medication Room** after reviewing the correct MAR.
- Click on **Unit Dosage** (or on the Unit Dosage cabinet); from the close-up view, click on drawer **201**.
- Select the medications you would like to administer. After each selection, click **Put Medication on Tray**. When you are finished selecting medications, click **Close Drawer** and then **View Medication Room**.
- Click **Automated System** (or on the Automated System unit itself). Click **Login**.
- On the next screen, specify the correct patient and drawer location.
- Select the medication you would like to administer and click **Put Medication on Tray**. Repeat this process if you wish to administer other medications from the Automated System.
- When you are finished, click **Close Drawer** and **View Medication Room**.
- From the Medication Room, click **Preparation** (or on the preparation tray).
- From the list of medications on your tray, highlight the correct medication to administer and click **Prepare**.
- This activates the Preparation Wizard. Supply any requested information; then click **Next**.
- Now select the correct patient to receive this medication and click **Finish**.
- Repeat the previous three steps until all medications that you want to administer are prepared.
- You can click on **Review Your Medications** and then on **Return to Medication Room** when ready. Once you are back in the Medication Room, go directly to Dorothy Grant's room by clicking on **201** at the bottom of the screen.
- Inside the patient's room, administer the medication, utilizing the six rights of medication administration. After you have collected the appropriate assessment data and are ready for administration, click **Patient Care** and then **Medication Administration**. Verify that the correct patient and medication(s) appear in the left-hand window. Highlight the first medication you wish to administer; then click the down arrow next to Select. From the drop-down menu, select **Administer** and complete the Administration Wizard by providing any information requested. When the Wizard stops asking for information, click **Administer to Patient**. Specify **Yes** when asked whether this administration should be recorded in the MAR. Finally, click **Finish**.

■ SELF-EVALUATION

Now let's see how you did during your medication administration!

- Click on **Leave the Floor** at the bottom of your screen. From the Floor Menu, select **Look at Your Preceptor's Evaluation**. Then click **Medication Scorecard**.

The following exercises will help you identify medication errors, investigate possible reasons for these errors, and reduce or prevent medication errors in the future.

1. Start by examining Table A. These are the medications you should have given to Dorothy Grant during this period of care. If each of the medications in Table A has a ✓ by it, then you made no errors. Congratulations!

If any medication has an X by it, then you made one or more medication errors.

Compare Tables A and B to determine which of the following types of errors you made: Wrong Dose, Wrong Route/Method/Site, or Wrong Time. Follow these steps:

a. Find medications in Table A that were given incorrectly.
b. Now see if those same medications are in Table B, which shows what you actually administered to Dorothy Grant.
c. Comparing Tables A and B, match the Strength, Dose, Route/Method/Site, and Time for each medication you administered incorrectly.
d. Then, using the form below, list the medications given incorrectly and mark the errors you made for each medication.

Medication	Strength	Dosage	Route	Method	Site	Time
	❑	❑	❑	❑	❑	❑
	❑	❑	❑	❑	❑	❑
	❑	❑	❑	❑	❑	❑
	❑	❑	❑	❑	❑	❑

2. To help you reduce future medication errors, consider the following list of possible reasons for errors.

   - Did not check drug against MAR for correct medication, correct dose, correct patient, correct route, correct time, correct documentation.
   - Did not check drug dose against MAR three times.
   - Did not open the unit dose package in the patient's room.
   - Did not correctly identify the patient using two identifiers.
   - Did not administer the drug on time.
   - Did not verify patient allergies.
   - Did not check the patient's current condition or vital sign parameters.
   - Did not consider why the patient would be receiving this drug.
   - Did not question why the drug was in the patient's drawer.
   - Did not check the physician's order and/or check with the pharmacist when there was a question about the drug or dose.
   - Did not verify that no adverse effects had occurred from a previous dose.

Based on the list of possibilities you just reviewed, determine how you made each error and record the reason in the form below:

Medication	Reason for Error

3. Look again at Table B. Are there medications listed that are not in Table A? If so, you gave a medication to Dorothy Grant that she should not have received. Complete the following exercises to help you understand how such an error might have been made.

   a. Perhaps you gave a medication that was on Dorothy Grant's MAR for this period of care, without recognizing that a change had occurred in the patient's condition, which should have caused you to reconsider. Review patient records as necessary and complete the following form:

Medication	Possible Reasons Not to Give This Medication

   b. Another possibility is that you gave Dorothy Grant a medication that should have been given at a different time. Check her MAR and complete the form below to determine whether you made a Wrong Time error:

Medication	Given to Dorothy Grant at What Time	Should Have Been Given at What Time

c. Maybe you gave another patient's medication to Dorothy Grant. In this case, you made a Wrong Patient error. Check the MARs of other patients and use the form below to determine whether you made this type of error:

Medication	Given to Dorothy Grant	Should Have Been Given to

4. The Medication Scorecard provides some other interesting sources of information. For example, if there is a medication selected for Dorothy Grant but it was not given to her, there will be an X by that medication in Table A, but it will not appear in Table B. In that case, you might have given this medication to some other patient, which is another type of Wrong Patient error. To investigate further, look at Table D, which lists the medications you gave to other patients. See whether you can find any medications ordered for Dorothy Grant that were given to another patient by mistake. However, before you make any decisions, be sure to cross-check the MAR for other patients because the same medication may have been ordered for multiple patients. Use the following form to record your findings:

Medication	Should Have Been Given to Dorothy Grant	Given by Mistake to

5. Now take some time to review the medication exercises you just completed. Use the form below to create an overall analysis of what you have learned. Once again, record each of the medication errors you made, including the type of each error. Then, for each error you made, indicate specifically what you would do differently to prevent this type of error from occurring again.

Medication	Type of Error	Error Prevention Tactic

Submit this form to your instructor if required as a graded assignment, or simply use these exercises to improve your understanding of medication errors and how to reduce them.

Name: ______________________ Date: ______________

The following icons are used throughout this workbook to help you quickly identify particular activities and assignments:

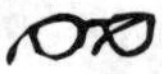 Indicates a reading assignment—tells you which textbook chapter(s) you should read before starting each lesson

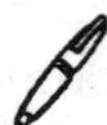 Indicates a writing activity

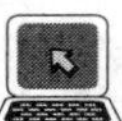 Marks the beginning of an interactive virtual hospital activity—signals you to open or return to your *Virtual Clinical Excursions—Obstetrics-Pediatrics* simulation

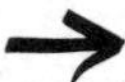 Indicates additional virtual hospital instructions

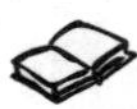 Indicates questions and activities that require you to consult your textbook

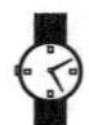 Indicates the approximate time required to complete an exercise

LESSON 1

The Childbearing and Child-Rearing Family

Reading Assignment: The Childbearing and Child-Rearing Family (Chapter 3)

Patients: Dorothy Grant, Room 201
Stacey Crider, Room 202
Kelly Brady, Room 203
Maggie Gardner, Room 204
Gabriela Valenzuela, Room 205
Laura Wilson, Room 206

Goal: Demonstrate an understanding of how the family, community, and culture affect the pregnant woman.

Objectives:

1. Assess and plan care for a patient from a specific culture.
2. Explore how your background influences the care that you give to patients who have differing experiences in regard to community, family, or culture.
3. Discuss the various types of families, communities, and cultures represented by each of the patients.

Exercise 1

Virtual Hospital Activity

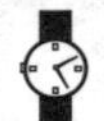

15 minutes

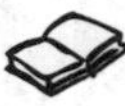

Review pages 38-41 in your textbook and complete the following exercise regarding family types.

Read question 1 before starting this period of care. Fill in the table as you review each patient's chart.

- Sign in to work at Pacific View Regional Hospital on the Obstetrics Floor for Period of Care 1. (*Note*: If you are already in the virtual hospital from a previous exercise, click on **Leave the Floor** and then on **Restart the Program** to get to the sign-in window.)
- From the Patient List, select all the patients to review.
- Click on **Go to Nurses' Station** and then on **Chart**.
- Click on **201** to open Dorothy Grant's chart.
- Click on **Admissions** and find the patient's marital status.
- Click on **History and Physical** and review the Family History section.
- Once you have completed the column for Dorothy Grant in the table below, click on **Return to Nurses' Station**.
- Click on **Chart** and then on **202** to open Stacey Crider's chart. Review to complete this patient's portion of the table below. Repeat this sequence until you have completed the table.

1. Under each patient's name below, place an X in the row that describes that patient's type of family. (*Note:* Some patients may require more than one X. Mark all descriptors that apply.)

	Dorothy Grant	**Stacey Crider**	**Kelly Brady**	**Maggie Gardner**	**Gabriela Valenzuela**	**Laura Wilson**
Traditional (nuclear)	X		X	X	X	
Single-parent						X
Multi-generational		X				
Blended						
High-risk	X		preeclampsia severe	X		X

2. Using what you learned in your chart review, along with the information in your textbook, identify the type of family that Gabriela Valenzuela has. Briefly describe how her family fits the type you have chosen.

3. Based on the information provided in your textbook, what type of family do you have? Describe how your family fits the description of the family type you have chosen.

Review pages 43-47 in your textbook regarding various cultural and religious groups.

4. Among the Asian-American culture, what is one form of medicine that is widely accepted? Give an example.

Herbal medicines and practices like acupressure. (p.46)

5. What do Native Americans believe in regard to health?

Health reflects living in total harmony with nature. (p.46)

6. What is one barrier in providing health care to patients from Middle Eastern cultures?
Obtaining a health history because Islam says family affairs are kept within the family (p.47)

7. In the Hispanic culture, religion and health are strongly associated. (p46)

8. Based on your review of the textbook reading, will you change your care for patients of differing cultures? If so, how? What community resources are available for patients of various cultures where you live?

Exercise 2

Virtual Hospital Activity

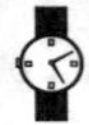

25 minutes

Culturally competent care is very important. As we review the various ways of providing culturally competent care, we will review two patients at Pacific View Regional Hospital.

- Sign in to work at Pacific View Regional Hospital on the Obstetrics Floor for Period of Care 1. (*Note*: If you are already in the virtual hospital from a previous exercise, click on **Leave the Floor** and then on **Restart the Program** to get to the sign-in window.)
- From the Patient List, select Stacey Crider and Maggie Gardner.
- Click on **Go to Nurses' Station**.
- Click on **Chart** and then on **202**.
- Click on **Nursing Admission** and review. (*Hint*: See the Role Relationships section.)

1. Identify a nursing diagnosis that would be appropriate for Stacey Crider and her family in regard to culture. Parents American-Indian, Husband Mexican strained relation b/t both

Maggie Gardner and her husband are very religious. According to the textbook, most members of the African-American culture have strong feelings about family, community, and religion. With this information in mind, complete the following activity and questions.

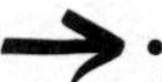

- Click on **Return to Nurses' Station**.
- Click on **204** at the bottom of the screen.
- Click on **Patient Care** and then on **Nurse-Client Interactions**.
- Select and view the video titled **0730: Communicating Empathy**. (*Note*: Check the virtual clock to see whether enough time has elapsed. You can use the fast-forward feature to advance the time by 2-minute intervals if the video is not yet available. Then click again on **Patient Care** and **Nurse-Client Interactions** to refresh the screen.)

2. What does Maggie Gardner's husband verbalize during this interaction that would correlate with the African-American population's deep sense of religion?

"I'm praying that we can just make it through this pregnancy"

3. Based on your interactions with patients in the hospital where you have worked, describe your experience(s) with caring for someone of a different culture. What are some of the ideals that are different from your own? What barriers to care have you experienced?

4. How comfortable are you with caring for patients from a different culture? Do you find yourself feeling judgmental or attempting to change others? What can you do to learn more about other cultures?

To further explore Jim and Maggie Gardner's spiritual perspective, return to the patient's chart.

- Click on **Chart** and then on **204**.
- Click on the **Consultations** and review the Pastoral Care Spiritual Assessment and the Pastoral Consultation.

5. What does Maggie Gardner "blame" her miscarriages on?

God is puishing her because she has harsh feelings towards her sister

6. What is Maggie Gardner's perception of God?

Powerful, loving, Kind. merciful, watching over, present, always there

7. What is one underlying theme that you see in the Consultations, Nursing Admission, and History and Physical sections of the chart in regard to religion and this patient's perception of her situation?

This pt. is very religious and

LESSON 2

Management of Fertility and Infertility

Reading Assignment: Reproductive Anatomy and Physiology (Chapter 11)
Management of Fertility and Infertility (Chapter 31)

Patients: Stacey Crider, Room 202
Kelly Brady, Room 203
Maggie Gardner, Room 204
Gabriela Valenzuela, Room 205
Laura Wilson, Room 206

Goal: Demonstrate an understanding of reproductive system concerns, contraception options, and infertility.

Objectives:

1. Identify reproductive concerns that can occur.
2. Differentiate among the varying types of contraception available.
3. Identify various methods of testing and treatment options that can be used for couples experiencing infertility concerns.

Exercise 1

Virtual Hospital Activity

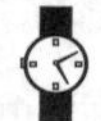

10 minutes

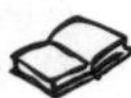

Review information on pages 200-209 in your textbook.

1. What is a normal length (or range) for a menstrual cycle?

2. What are the criteria required to diagnose an individual with amenorrhea?

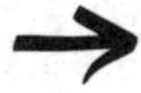

- Sign in to work at Pacific View Regional Hospital on the Obstetrics Floor for Period of Care 1. (*Note*: If you are already in the virtual hospital from a previous exercise, click on **Leave the Floor** and then on **Restart the Program** to get to the sign-in window.)
- From the Patient List, select Stacey Crider.
- Click on **Go to Nurses' Station**.
- Click on **Chart** and then on **202**.
- Click on **History and Physical** and review the patient's gynecologic history. (*Hint:* See the bottom of page 1.)

3. Does Stacey Crider meet the textbook criteria for amenorrhea?

4. What is her history?

5. List three things that can cause the disruption of ovulation. (*Hint:* See pages 755-756 in your textbook.)

Exercise 2

Virtual Hospital Activity

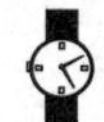

20 minutes

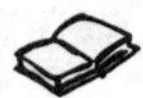

Review pages 736-754 in your textbook.

1. What is contraception?

2. What is the primary focus of counseling when recommending/evaluating methods of contraception?

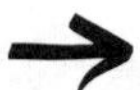

- Sign in to work at Pacific View Regional Hospital on the Obstetrics Floor for Period of Care 1. (*Note*: If you are already in the virtual hospital from a previous exercise, click on **Leave the Floor** and then on **Restart the Program** to get to the sign-in window.)
- From the Patient List, select Kelly Brady, Gabriela Valenzuela, and Laura Wilson.
- Click on **Go to Nurses' Station**.
- Click on **Chart** and then on **203** for Kelly Brady's chart.
- Review the **History and Physical**.
- Repeat the previous three steps for Gabriela Valenzuela (205) and Laura Wilson (206).

3. Identify the birth control method each woman was using before her current pregnancy.

Kelly Brady

Gabriela Valenzuela

Laura Wilson

4. Gabriela Valenzuela is Catholic. Which method of birth control would be appropriate for the nurse to discuss with her?

5. What does this method rely on?

6. Kelly Brady wants to use oral contraceptives while breastfeeding to prevent pregnancy. Which type of oral contraception is appropriate for her to use? Why?

7. Laura Wilson is HIV-positive. What is the most appropriate form of birth control for her? Why?

Exercise 3

Virtual Hospital Activity

20 minutes

Review pages 754-767 in your textbook.

1. __________% of women of reproductive age have a problem with infertility.

2. When a woman reaches her ____________________, a natural decline in fertility begins.

3. List four factors that affect male fertility.

4. List at least three factors that affect female fertility.

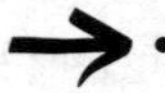

- Sign in to work at Pacific View Regional Hospital on the Obstetrics Floor for Period of Care 1. (*Note*: If you are already in the virtual hospital from a previous exercise, click on **Leave the Floor** and then on **Restart the Program** to get to the sign-in window.)
- From the Patient List, select Maggie Gardner.
- Click on **Go to Nurses' Station**.
- Click on **Chart** and then on **204**.
- Review the **History and Physical**.

5. Maggie Gardner was married __________ years before she conceived the first time.

6. Based on the textbook reading, which of the following would Maggie Gardner have been diagnosed with if she had chosen to get treatment after 1 year of attempting to get pregnant?
   a. Primary infertility
   b. Secondary infertility

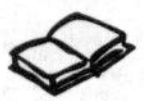

Review pages 758-762 in your textbook to answer the following questions.

7. List at least three tests that can be completed on a male patient to determine the causes of infertility.

8. List at least four tests can be completed on a female patient to determine the causes of infertility.

9. What test is used to assess a couple to determine adequacy of cervical mucus and sperm function after sexual intercourse has occurred?

10. What methods are available to assist an infertile couple to conceive?

11. Which methods did Maggie Gardner and her husband use to assist in getting pregnant? (*Hint*: Review the OB history in the History and Physical.)

LESSON 3

Nutrition for Childbearing/ Prenatal Diagnostic Tests

Reading Assignment: Nutrition for Childbearing (Chapter 14)
Prenatal Diagnostic Tests (Chapter 15)
Concurrent Disorders During Pregnancy (Chapter 26)

Patients: Kelly Brady, Room 203
Maggie Gardner, Room 204

Goal: Demonstrate an understanding of the assessment of risk factors in pregnancy, including maternal and fetal nutritional aspects.

Objectives:

1. Identify appropriate interventions for maintaining adequate maternal and fetal nutrition.
2. Differentiate among the varying types of assessment techniques that can be used with both low- and high-risk pregnancy patients.
3. Identify various methods of testing that can be used in high-risk pregnancies.

Exercise 1

Virtual Hospital Activity

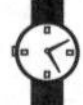

15 minutes

- Sign in to work at Pacific View Regional Hospital on the Obstetrics Floor for Period of Care 1. (*Note*: If you are already in the virtual hospital from a previous exercise, click on **Leave the Floor** and then on **Restart the Program** to get to the sign-in window.)
- From the Patient List, select Maggie Gardner
- Click on **Go to Nurses' Station**.
- Click on **Chart** and then on **204**.
- Click on **Laboratory Reports**.

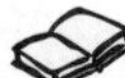

Review information regarding anemia on pages 291-292 and 621-623 in your textbook.

normal hematocrit: at least 33% 1st & 3rd tri, at least 32% 2nd tri
normal hemoglobin: at least 11g/dL 1st & 3rd tri, at least 10.5g/dL 2nd tri

1. What were Maggie Gardner's hemoglobin and hematocrit levels on admission?

hemoglobin: 9.6

hematocrit: 31

→ • Click on **History and Physical**.

2. What puts Maggie Gardner at a greater risk for developing anemia than the average pregnant patient? (*Hint*: Review the Genetic Screening section of her History and Physical.)

- Sickle cell disease or trait

3. What complication(s) do women with anemia experience at a higher rate than those without anemia?

- more susceptible to infection, ↑ chance of preeclampsia - eclampsia and postpartal hemorrhage

4. What is a normal hematocrit level for a woman who is pregnant?

at least 33% in 1st and 3rd trimester
at least 32% in 2nd trimester

5. What assessments, specifically related to an anemia diagnosis, need to be performed by the nurse at each prenatal visit?

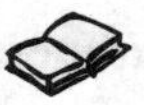

6. According to your textbook, what are some good sources of iron that you could instruct Maggie Gardner to add to her diet? (P621)

Meat, fish, Chicken, and green leafy vegetables.

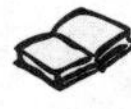

7. Maggie Gardner is not on iron supplementation at this time; however, list at least three things that you could teach her about iron supplementation.

(P621)
- less gastrointestinal discomfort if taken with meals
- taking 500mg of vit C may help absorption
- Therapy often continued for 6 months after anemia is corrected

Exercise 2

Virtual Hospital Activity

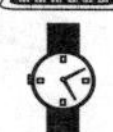

15 minutes

- Sign in to work at Pacific View Regional Hospital on the Obstetrics Floor for Period of Care 3. (*Note*: If you are already in the virtual hospital from a previous exercise, click on **Leave the Floor** and then on **Restart the Program** to get to the sign-in window.)
- From the Patient List, select Maggie Gardner.
- Click on **Go to Nurses' Station**.
- Click on **Chart** and then on **204**.
- Click on **Diagnostic Reports**.

Review information regarding ultrasounds on pages 301-304 in your textbook.

1. List at least three things that ultrasounds are used for during the first trimester. (P.303)

- Determin presence & location of pregnancy
- Determin multifetal gestations
- Identify the need for follow-up testing

2. List at least three things that ultrasounds are used for during the second and third trimesters. (p 303)

-Evaluate fetal anatomy
-Assess progress of fetal growth
-Determine fetal presentation

3. What are two forms of ultrasound? When is each form used?

Transvaginal ultrasound is used during 1st trimester
Transabdominal ultrasound is used during 2nd + 3rd trimester

4. What type of ultrasound is Maggie Gardner having?

5. Based on the ultrasound findings, how large is her baby?

1200g

6. List three abnormalities found on the ultrasound in regard to the placenta.

- Partial placenta previa present
- Placenta grade II with multiple calcification & infarcts noted in placenta
- Some larger indentations extend down toward the uterine wall
- Comma-like & basal echogenic densities noted

7. What is the impression from Maggie Gardner's ultrasound in terms of the fetus and the placenta?

- No fetal anomalies noted
- Need furter study to determine adequacy of placental function
- Multiple areas of calcification & infarctions noted

8. What are the recommendations regarding follow-up?

- Serial ultrasound to monitor placental function
- Doppler studies may be indicated

Exercise 3

Virtual Hospital Activity

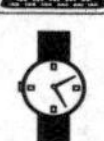

15 minutes

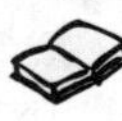

Biophysical profile is another very important assessment tool used with patients who are experiencing a high-risk pregnancy. Review information regarding biophysical profiles on pages 311-313 in your textbook.

1. What five markers are assessed on a biophysical profile? (*Hint:* See Table 15-1 in your textbook.) (313)

- Nonstress test (NST)
- Fetal breathing movements (FBM)
- Gross body movements
- Fetal tone
- Amniotic Fluid volume

2. The amount of amniotic fluid provides information about long-term hypoxia.
(P312)

3. Normal values for each of the markers listed in question 1 suggest adequate nerological function and oxygenation.

4. Below, list the markers that are considered acute and those that are considered chronic.
(P311)

Acute markers
- FHR reactivity
- Fetal breathing movements
- Gross body movements
- Fetal tone

Chronic markers
- the volume of amniotic fluid

- Sign in to work at Pacific View Regional Hospital on the Obstetrics Floor for Period of Care 3. (*Note*: If you are already in the virtual hospital from a previous exercise, click on **Leave the Floor** and then on **Restart the Program** to get to the sign-in window.)
- From the Patient List, select Kelly Brady.
- Click on **Go to Nurses' Station**.
- Click on **Chart** and then on **203**.
- Click on **Diagnostic Reports**.

5. What is the estimated gestational age of Kelly Brady's fetus?
26 2/7 weeks

6. What is the amniotic fluid index as indicated on the report?
12.9

7. Suppose that Kelly Brady had an abnormally low amount of amniotic fluid. What might this indicate?
Low amount indicates prolonged fetal hypoxia and possible fetal compromise

8. What is the normal amniotic fluid index value? (p313)
Volume sums greater than 10 cm are

9. What is Kelly Brady's score on the biophysical profile?
10/10

10. Based on the information you have reviewed in your textbook, what does this score indicate?

LESSON 4

Pain Management for Childbirth

Reading Assignment: Pain Management for Childbirth (Chapter 18)

Patients: Kelly Brady, Room 203
Gabriela Valenzuela, Room 205
Laura Wilson, Room 206

Goal: Demonstrate an understanding of the normal labor and birth process.

Objectives:

1. Assess and identify factors that influence pain perception.
2. Describe selected nonpharmacologic and pharmacologic measures for pain management during labor and birth.

Exercise 1

Virtual Hospital Activity

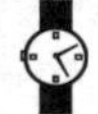

45 minutes

- Sign in to work at Pacific View Regional Hospital on the Obstetrics Floor for Period of Care 1. (*Note*: If you are already in the virtual hospital from a previous exercise, click on **Leave the Floor** and then on **Restart the Program** to get to the sign-in window.)
- From the Patient List, select Laura Wilson.
- Click on **Get Report**.

1. What is Laura Wilson's current condition, according to the change-of-shift report?

- easily awakened for vital signs & assessments
- resting comfortably
- no uterine contractions
- positive fetal movement
- denies nausea or abdominal pain

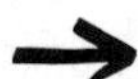

- Click on **Go to Nurses' Station**.
- Click on **206** at the bottom of the screen.
- Read the Initial Observations.

2. What is your impression of Laura Wilson's condition?

same as Q#1

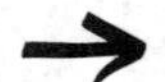

- Click on **Patient Care** and then on **Nurse-Client Interactions**.
- Select and view the video titled **0730: Patient Assessment**. (*Note*: Check the virtual clock to see whether enough time has elapsed. You can use the fast-forward feature to advance the time by 2-minute intervals if the video is not yet available. Then click again on **Patient Care** and **Nurse-Client Interactions** to refresh the screen.)

3. What is Laura Wilson's assessment of her current condition? How does this compare with the information you received from the shift report and the Initial Observations summary?

Laura states she has stomach pain, and is a little sick to her stomach

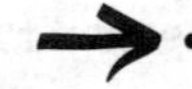

- Click on **Chart** and then on **206**.
- Click on **Nursing Admission**.

4. List Laura Wilson's admission diagnoses. (*Hint:* See page 1 of the Nursing Admission form.)

- High-risk pregnancy at 37 weeks
- HIV + with vomiting, diarrhea and fever
- Past IV drug use
- Current marijuana and crack cocaine use

5. What is your perception of Laura Wilson's behavior? What data did you collect during this exercise that led you to this perception?

6. Think about the following questions and then discuss your ideas with your classmates: Do your personal values and beliefs contribute to your perception of Laura Wilson's behavior? If so, how? What nursing interventions might help to overcome your personal biases when dealing with Laura Wilson?

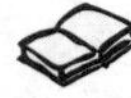 Read the section on factors influencing pain response on pages 389-391 in your textbook.

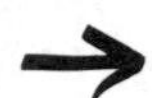
- Continue reviewing Laura Wilson's **Nursing Admission** form as needed to answer question 7.

7. Each woman's pain during childbirth is unique and is influenced by a variety of factors. For each factor listed below and on the next page, explain how that factor influences pain perception (in the middle column). In the right column, list data from Laura Wilson's Nursing Admission that support how that factor might relate to her particular pain perception.

Factor	Typical Effect on Pain Perception	Laura Wilson's Supporting Data
Anxiety	- magnifys sensitivity to pain and impairs the ability to tolerate it	
Previous experience	- A woman's natural reaction to pain during labor is fear and withdrawal	

Factor	Typical Effect on Pain Perception	Laura Wilson's Supporting Data
Childbirth preparation	-Preparation reduces anxiety and Fear of the unknown -Allows woman to rehearse for labor and learn skills to master pain as labor progresses	-She wanted to sign up for childbirth preparation classes, but never did
Support	-an axious partner or other support is less able to provide the encouragement & reassurance the woman needs -anxiety in others can be contagious, and an anxious partner can ↑ woman's anxiety	-parent's want baby to be put up for adoption -boyfrient is out of town

Exercise 2

Virtual Hospital Activity

45 minutes

- Sign in to work at Pacific View Regional Hospital on the Obstetrics Floor for Period of Care 2. (*Note*: If you are already in the virtual hospital from a previous exercise, click on **Leave the Floor** and then on **Restart the Program** to get to the sign-in window.)
- From the Patient List, select Gabriela Valenzuela.

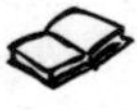

Read the sections on Cutaneous Stimulation, Mental Stimulation, and Breathing (pages 392-395) in your textbook.

1. Cutaneous stimulation includes self-massage, massage by others, Thermal stimulation, and acupressure. Touch can communicate caring, comfort, affirmation, and reassurance.

2. Breathing techniques provide a different focus during contractions, interfering with pain sensory transmission. The woman should begin with simple breathing patterns and progress to more complex ones as greater distraction is needed. Each contraction begins and ends with a cleansing breath. The cleansing breath helps the woman release tension and focus on relaxing, provides oxygen, and signals her labor partner that the contraction is beginning or ending.

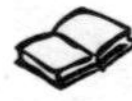
Now read the section on Pharmacologic Pain Management for Labor on pages 395-410 in your textbook.

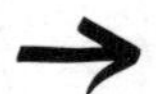
- Click on **Get Report** and review this report.

3. Is Gabriela Valenzuela in labor at this time? Give a rationale for your answer.

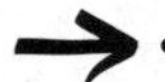
- Click on **Go to Nurses' Station**.
- Click on **205** at the bottom of the screen.
- Click on **Patient Care** and then on **Nurse-Client Interactions**.
- Select and view the video titled **1140: Intervention—Bleeding, Comfort**. (*Note*: Check the virtual clock to see whether enough time has elapsed. You can use the fast-forward feature to advance the time by 2-minute intervals if the video is not yet available. Then click again on **Patient Care** and **Nurse-Client Interactions** to refresh the screen.)
- After viewing the video, click on **Chart** and then on **205**.
- Click on **Nurse's Notes**.
- Scroll to the entry for 1140 on Wednesday.

4. How is Gabriela Valenzuela tolerating labor at this time?

Gabriela is complaining of increased pain with contractions

5. What pain interventions does the nurse implement at this time?

The nures provides fentanyl, asks husband to coach through breathing and rub her back

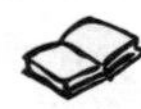
In your textbook, read about fentanyl in Table 18-1 and in the section on Systemic Drugs for Labor on pages 400-402.

6. What is the action of this drug?

Inhibits ascending pain pathways in CNS, increases pain threshold

Let's begin the process for preparing and administering Gabriela Valenzuela's fentanyl dose.

- First, click on **Return to Room 205** and then on **Medication Room**.
- Next, click on **MAR** and then on tab **205**.
- Scroll down to the PRN Medication Administration Record for Wednesday.

7. What is the ordered dose of fentanyl?

50mcg IV every 30-60min prn pain, max 600mcg /24hr

- Click on **Return to Medication Room**.
- Click on **Automated System**.
- Click on **Login**.
- In box 1, click on **Gabriela Valenzuela, 205**.
- In box 2, click on **Automated System Drawer A-F**.
- Click on **Fentanyl citrate**.
- Click on **Put Medication on Tray**.
- Click on **Close Drawer**.
- Click on **View Medication Room**.
- Click on **Preparation**.
- Click on **Prepare** and follow the Preparation Wizard prompts to complete preparation of Gabriela Valenzuela's fentanyl dose. When the Wizard stops requesting information, click **Finish**.
- Click on **Return to Medication Room**.
- Click on **205** to go to the patient's room.

8. What additional assessments must be completed before you administer Gabriela Valenzuela's medication?

- Vital signs
- respiratory status
- CNS changes
- Allergic reaction

9. Why is it important to check Gabriela Valenzuela's respirations before giving the dose of fentanyl?

Fentanyl can decrese respirations.

10. What safety precautions should be in effect for Gabriela Valenzuela after she receives this dose of fentanyl?

bed rails up, monitor resp. status, monitor responce to fentanyl

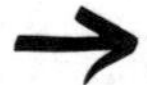

- Click on **Patient Care** and then on **Medication Administration**.
- Click on **Review Your Medications** and verify the accuracy of your preparation. Click on **Return to Room 205**.
- Next, click the down arrow next to **Select** and choose **Administer**.
- Follow the Administration Wizard prompts to administer Gabriela Valenzuela's fentanyl dose. (*Note:* Click **Yes** when asked whether to document this administration in the MAR.)
- When the Wizard stops asking questions, click on **Finish**.
- Still in Gabriela Valenzuela's room, click on **Patient Care** and then on **Nurse-Client Interactions**.
- Select and view the video titled **1155: Evaluation—Comfort Measures**. (*Note*: Check the virtual clock to see whether enough time has elapsed. You can use the fast-forward feature to advance the time by 2-minute intervals if the video is not yet available. Then click again on **Patient Care** and **Nurse-Client Interactions** to refresh the screen.)

11. How effective were the interventions you identified in question 5?

The interventions were effective she rates her pain 2-3/10

Read the section on Helping the Woman Use Nonpharmacologic Techniques on pages 406-407 in your textbook.

12. Gabriela Valenzuela is most likely experiencing hyperventilation. Other symptoms of hyperventilation include dizziness, tingling and numbness of the fingers and lips and carpopedal spasm.

13. What interventions does the nurse suggest to deal with this problem? List other interventions described in your textbook.

Not to breath to fast which can make her feel dizzy

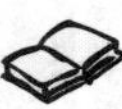 At the end of the 1155 video, Gabriela Valenzuela states that she “doesn’t want any needles” in her back. Learn more about this by reading the section on Epidural Block on pages 396-400 in your textbook.

14. What could you tell Gabriela Valenzuela to help her make an informed decision about anesthesia for labor? In the table below, list advantages and disadvantages of epidural anesthesia.

Advantages	Disadvantages
-Relieves discomfort during labor and birth	-Maternal hypotension
-Woman is fully awake and a part of the birth process	-Labor progress and fetal decent may be slowed
-Continuous epidural allows different blocking for each stages of labor	-Pushing efforts in second stage may be less effetive due to decreased sensation
-Many times the woman's urge to bear down is preserved	-Length of labor is increased by approximately 25 mins
	-Delay in return of bladder sensation may result

Before leaving this period of care, let’s see how you did preparing and administering the patient’s medication.

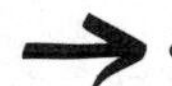

- Click on **Leave the Floor**.
- Click on **Look at Your Preceptor’s Evaluation**.
- Click on **Medication Scorecard** and review the evaluation. How did you do? (*Hint:* For a quick refresher on reading your Medication Scorecard, see page 22 in the **Getting Started** section of this workbook. For a more detailed tour on preparing and administering medications and interpreting your scorecard, see pages 26-30 and 37-41.)

Exercise 3

Virtual Hospital Activity

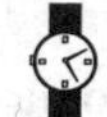

20 minutes

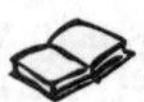

Read the section on General Anesthesia on pages 402-403 in your textbook.

- Sign in to work at Pacific View Regional Hospital on the Obstetrics Floor for Period of Care 4. (*Note*: If you are already in the virtual hospital from a previous exercise, click on **Leave the Floor** and then on **Restart the Program** to get to the sign-in window.)
- From the Nurses' Station, click on **Chart** and then on **203** for Kelly Brady's chart. (*Remember:* You are not able to visit patients or administer medications during Period of Care 4. You are able to review patient records only.)
- Click on **Nurse's Notes**.
- Scroll to the entry for 1730 on Wednesday.

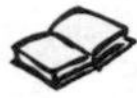

1. Why does the anesthesiologist plan to use general anesthesia during Kelly Brady's cesarean section? (*Hint*: Read the section on Contraindications and Precautions on pages 397-398 in your textbook.)

Contraindications: refusal, coagulation defects, uncorrected hypovolemia, an infection in the area of insetion or a severe systemic infection, allergy, fetal condition that demands birth sooner than the block can become effective

The anesthesiologist plans on general anesthesia due to Kelly Brady's low platelet count

2. Why is Kelly Brady upset about receiving general anesthesia for her surgery?

She wanted to be awake so she could see her baby as soon as she is born.

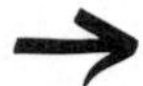

- Click on **Physician's Orders**.
- Review the entry for Wednesday at 1540.

3. What preoperative medications are ordered for Kelly Brady?

- Sodium citrate 500mg / citric acid 334 mg solution 30mL PO
- metoclopramide hydrochloride
- ranitidine hydrochloride

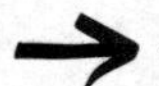

- Click on **Return to Nurses' Station**.
- Click on the **Drug** icon in the lower left corner of your screen to access the Drug Guide.
- Use the search box or the scroll bar to read about each of the drugs you listed in question 3.

4. All of these medications are given preoperatively to help prevent aspiration pneumonia. Using information from the Drug Guide and from the section on General Anesthesia in your textbook, match each of the medications below with the description of how it specifically works to prevent aspiration pneumonia.

	Medication	How It Prevents Aspiration Pneumonia
c	Sodium citrate/citric acid (Bicitra)	a. Decreases the production of gastric acid
b	Metoclopramide (Reglan)	b. Prevents nausea and vomiting and accelerates gastric emptying
a	Ranitidine (Zantac)	c. Raises the gastric pH to neutralize acidic stomach contents

5. How would you expect general anesthesia to affect Kelly Brady's baby? Why?

The general anesthesia can cause resp. depression in the baby if delivery after starting anesthesia is delayed

LESSON 5

The Childbearing Family with Special Needs: Adolescent Pregnancy, Delayed Pregnancy, and Substance Abuse

Reading Assignment: The Childbearing Family with Special Needs (Chapter 24, pages 550-563)

Patients: Laura Wilson, Room 206
Kelly Brady, Room 203

Goal: Demonstrate an understanding of the special needs of pregnant adolescents, mature primigravidas, and women with substance abuse issues.

Objectives:

1. Describe differences in the normal pregnancy changes experienced by adolescent and older mothers.
2. Assess and plan care for a substance-abusing woman with a term pregnancy.

Exercise 1

Virtual Hospital Activity

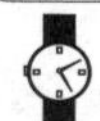

20 minutes

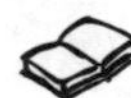

Laura Wilson and Kelly Brady represent age extremes among women of childbearing age. First, read the section on Adolescent Pregnancy on pages 550-556 in your textbook.

1. Despite recent decreases, the pregnancy and birth rates for teenagers in the United States are higher________ than those in other developed countries. About 82%________ of teen pregnancies are unintended. 19___% of pregnant adolescents have had 1 or more________ previous births.

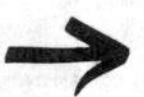

- Sign in to work at Pacific View Regional Hospital on the Obstetrics Floor for Period of Care 4. (*Note*: If you are already in the virtual hospital from a previous exercise, click on **Leave the Floor** and then on **Restart the Program** to get to the sign-in window.)
- From the Nurses' Station, click on **Chart** and then on **206**. (*Remember:* You are not able to visit patients or administer medications during Period of Care 4. You are able to review patient records only.)
- Click on **Nursing Admission**.

2. The table below and on the next page lists several common characteristics of pregnant adolescents, according to your textbook. Based on information found in the Nursing Admission, explain how each of these characteristics applies (or does not apply) to Laura Wilson.

Characteristic	Laura Wilson's Data
Pregnancy unintended	unplanned
Inadequate or no prenatal care	prenatal care started at 20 weeks
Smoker	10-20 per day
Inadequate weight gain	gained 22 pounds with pregnancy
Unmarried	Single

Characteristic	Laura Wilson's Data
Not ready for emotional, psychologic, and financial responsibilities of parenthood	-If parents stop paying rent wouldn't be able to aford food. -Not sure how to manage baby at home with no help -unrealistic and inadequate plans for future
High incidence of sexually transmitted diseases	HIV positive

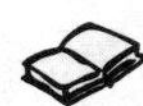 Now read the section on Delayed Pregnancy on pages 556-558 in your textbook.

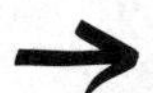

- Click on **Return to Nurses' Station**.
- Click on **Chart** and then on **203** for Kelly Brady's chart.
- Click on **Nursing Admission**.

3. The table below and on the next page lists several common characteristics of mature primigravidas. Based on the information found in the Nursing Admission, explain how each of these characteristics applies (or does not apply) to Kelly Brady.

Characteristic	Kelly Brady's Data
Pregnancy delayed to pursue a career or for financial reasons	
Decision to become pregnant made after careful thought	-Put off having children until they were ready

Characteristic	Kelly Brady's Data
Usually has financial security, a stable relationship, and personal maturity	- Works full-time in a demanding, responcible joby - in a relationship with husband
Often adopts health-promoting activities	- Stopped all alcohol intake when began trying to conceive
Receptive to education on childbearing and/or child-rearing topics; likely to seek out information from a variety of sources	- plans on taking child birthing classes
Concerned about complications that may affect the fetus or own health	- worried about her baby and how preclampsia will affect her baby

4. Preeclampsia and gestational diabetes occur more frequently in the older gravida.
   a. True (circled)
   b. False

5. The risk for multiple birth (twins, triplets, etc.) decreases with advanced maternal age.
   a. True
   b. False (circled)

Exercise 2

Virtual Hospital Activity

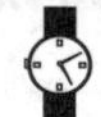

20 minutes

- Sign in to work at Pacific View Regional Hospital on the Obstetrics Floor for Period of Care 2. (*Note*: If you are already in the virtual hospital from a previous exercise, click on **Leave the Floor** and then on **Restart the Program** to get to the sign-in window.)
- From the Patient List, select Laura Wilson.
- Click on **Go to Nurses' Station**.
- Click on **Chart** and then on **206**.
- Click on **Nursing Admission**.

1. Based on your review of the Nursing Admission, complete the table below by documenting Laura Wilson's use of alcohol and recreational drugs.

Substance	Reported Use
Tobacco 10-20 per day	
Alcohol none to several per week	
* Marijuana few times a week	
* Crack cocaine Occasionally from 0 to several per week	

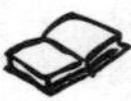 Read about the maternal and fetal effects of tobacco, alcohol, marijuana, and cocaine in the Substance Abuse section on pages 558-560 and Table 24-1 in your textbook.

2. For each pregnancy-related risk listed in the table below, place an X under the substance(s) thought to be associated with that risk.

Maternal or Fetal Effect	Tobacco	Alcohol	Marijuana	Cocaine
Spontaneous abortion	X	X		X
Premature rupture of membranes	X			X
Preterm labor	X			X
Decreased placental perfusion	X			
Abruptio placentae	X	X		X
Fetal alcohol syndrome (FAS)		X		
Fetal alcohol effects (FAE)		X		
Hypertension				X
Fetal demise		X		
Fetal anomalies			X	
Increased risk for sudden infant death syndrome (SIDS)	X			
Fetal growth restriction		X		
Prematurity	X			X

- Click on **Return to Nurses' Station**.
- Click on **206** at the bottom of the screen.
- Click on **Patient Care** and then on **Nurse-Client Interactions**.
- Select and view the video titled **1115: Teaching—Effects of Drug Use**. (*Note*: Check the virtual clock to see whether enough time has elapsed. You can use the fast-forward feature to advance the time by 2-minute intervals if the video is not yet available. Then click again on **Patient Care** and **Nurse-Client Interactions** to refresh the screen.)

3. Does Laura Wilson consider herself to be addicted? Support your answer with comments from the video.

No She stated that she can quit any time

4. How does Laura Wilson think her drug use will affect her baby?

She thinks that the baby can't be affected if its just one time.

5. According to the nurse in the video, how might Laura Wilson's drug use affect the baby?

- Cocaine can cause long term growth and development proplems
- the baby could go through withdrawal

Read the section on Interventions on pages 561-563 in your textbook.

6. Assume that you are the nurse caring for Laura Wilson today. Which interventions would be most appropriate to deal with Laura Wilson's drug use at this time? Select all that apply.

 X Talk with Laura Wilson in a manner that conveys caring and concern.

 X Urge Laura Wilson to begin a drug treatment program today.

_____ Explain to Laura Wilson that she may lose custody of her baby if her drug use continues.

_____ Involve other members of the health care team in Laura Wilson's care.

7. Explain your choice(s) in question 6.

2 because laura wants to be a good mom and has stated that she wants to quit for the baby

1 because convaying care and concerne may encourage laura to open so s

LESSON 6

The Childbearing Family with Special Needs: Pregnancy Loss and Intimate Partner Violence

Reading Assignment: The Childbearing Family with Special Needs (Chapter 24, pages 563-573)

Patients: Dorothy Grant, Room 201
Maggie Gardner, Room 204

Goals: Demonstrate an understanding of the grieving process and how it relates to coping with a current pregnancy. Identify patients at risk for intimate partner violence (IPV), interventions to assist those at risk, and ways to educate and empower those individuals toward healthy relationships.

Objectives:

1. Identify the various types of loss as they relate to a pregnancy.
2. Identify various methods of coping exhibited by patients who have experienced the loss of a newborn.
3. Discuss the statistics related to IPV.
4. List characteristics of battered women.
5. Explore the myths and facts regarding IPV.
6. Identify the nurse's role in regard to battered women or those involved in IPV.

Exercise 1

Writing Activity

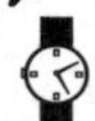

15 minutes

1. Parents may grieve not only the death of a newborn but also the birth of a baby with a reparable defect or irreparable defect.

2. What emotions do parents experience with multifetal pregnancy loss and the concurrent survival of one or more of the infants? How does this affect the grieving process?

- Parents experience conflicting and complex feelings of joy and grief. They may also experience fear about the health of the surviving one and may have problems with attachment.
- They may be unable to grieve for the dead child due to concerns for the surviving child

3. What potential problems may a previous pregnancy loss cause in a woman experiencing a subsequent pregnancy?

The women may have higher levels of anxiety, symptoms of depression, pessimistic about the chance of success and may be fearful near the time of previous pregnancy loss

4. All women and men who undergo a loss receive the support that they need.
   a. True
   b. False

Exercise 2

Virtual Hospital Activity

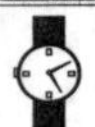

10 minutes

- Sign in to work at Pacific View Regional Hospital on the Obstetrics Floor for Period of Care 4. (*Note*: If you are already in the virtual hospital from a previous exercise, click on **Leave the Floor** and then on **Restart the Program** to get to the sign-in window.)
- Click on **Chart** and then on **204** for Maggie Gardner's chart. (*Remember:* You are not able to visit patients or administer medications during Period of Care 4. You are able to review patient records only.)
- Review the **History and Physical**.

1. How many losses related to pregnancy has Maggie Gardner experienced?

6 pregnancy losses

- Click on **Nursing Admission**.

2. What is the first evidence you find that Maggie Gardner's previous losses are affecting her current pregnancy and care? (*Hint*: Review the first five sections of the Nursing Admission.)

Has not kept several appointments. She states she's ~~worried~~ afraid she will find out something is wrong.

→ • Click on **Consultations**.

3. To what does Maggie Gardner attribute her inability to have a child?

Maggie believes God must be punishing her ~~for something she has done~~ because of her harsh feelings towards her sister

4. List three therapeutic measures the chaplain can use to assist Maggie Gardner through these feelings as part of her grieving process.

- Explore perceptions
- Explore relationship with God and others
- Provide comfort

5. What did the chaplain accomplish during his time with Maggie Gardner?

The chaplain discussed coping mechanisms to be utilized with various stressors.

6. Acknowledging the deceased infant is extremely important in helping the parents work through their loss. What are the rights of the baby that may help the parents through the grieving process?

7. Now that you have read the information regarding the grieving process, let's explore your experiences. Have you ever suffered a loss or taken care of a patient who had just experienced a loss? What emotions did you experience or perceive from that patient? What responses did you communicate to the patient? Were they therapeutic? How might you have handled it differently?

Exercise 3

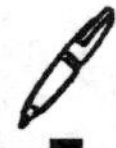

Writing Activity

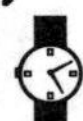

15 minutes

1. Match each statistic with the description to which it applies.

	Description	Statistic
d	Number of women abused that abuse their children	a. 25%
a	Percentage of women who report IPV at some point in their lives	b. Up to 20%
c	Percentage of homes where IPV has occurred in which children are also abused	c. 33% to 77%
b	Estimated percentage of women who are victims of IPV during pregnancy	d. 27%
e	Number of acts of IPV occurring to women	e. 4.8 million per year

Abuse of women has been common throughout history. Unfortunately, this continues today. Based on information from your textbook, answer true or false to the following questions.

2. IPV may start or increase in frequency and severity during pregnancy and the postpartum period.
   a. True
   b. False

3. Physical abuse during pregnancy may result in maternal or fetal death.
   a. True
   b. False

4. Substance abuse is often associated with physical abuse.
   a. True
   b. False

5. Physical violence is limited to hitting and slapping.
   a. True
   b. False

6. Children who are abused are more likely to become abusive as adults compared with children who have never been abused.
   a. True
   b. False

7. An abusive man often attempts to control all aspect of the woman's life.

Exercise 4

Virtual Hospital Activity

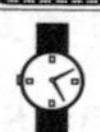

15 minutes

- Sign in to work at Pacific View Regional Hospital on the Obstetrics Floor for Period of Care 1. (*Note*: If you are already in the virtual hospital from a previous exercise, click on **Leave the Floor** and then on **Restart the Program** to get to the sign-in window.)
- From the Patient List, select Dorothy Grant.
- Click on Go to **Nurses' Station**.
- Click on **Chart** and select **201**.
- Click on **Nursing Admission**.

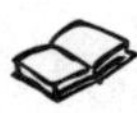

Review the Nursing Admission for Dorothy Grant's perspective of the abusive relationship that she has experienced. Also review pages 568-573 in your textbook.

1. What is the reality of Dorothy Grant's situation? How does that correlate with the textbook reading?

-She fears husband
-Husband makes all decisions
-She has low self-esteem
-Limited social interactions
-She doesn't work

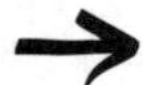

- Click on **Return to Nurses' Station**.
- Click on **201** at the bottom of the screen.
- Click on the **Patient Care** and then on **Nurse-Client Interactions**.
- Select and view the video titled **0810: Monitoring/Patient Support**. (*Note*: Check the virtual clock to see whether enough time has elapsed. You can use the fast-forward feature to advance the time by 2-minute intervals if the video is not yet available. Then click again on **Patient Care** and **Nurse-Client Interactions** to refresh the screen.)

2. In the video interaction, what does Dorothy Grant say she should do to help prevent the violence?

-Keep kids safe

- thougt did more or tried harder

3. In the video, what are Dorothy Grant's current concerns?

-She is worried about delivering baby early

- Click on **Go to Nurses' Station**.
- Click on **Chart** and then on **201**.
- Click on **Consultations** and review the Psychiatric Consult and the Social Work Consult.

Review the information regarding the myths and realities about IPV on page 570 in your textbook. Based on that information and your review of Dorothy Grant's chart, answer the following questions.

4. Dorothy Grant stays in the relationship because of ______________ and ______________________________.

5. The percentage of women who are battered during pregnancy is up to 20%.

6. Based on the information provided, in what phase of the abuse cycle is Dorothy Grant?

7. According to the consults, Dorothy Grant has several options. What are some of the options that the social worker and psychiatric heath care provider can offer her or assist her with?

- Offer support & encouragement in making a change in her life

- Explore with patient restraining order againt husband

- Discuss battered women's shelter placement

8. Dorothy Grant's husband blames her for the pregnancy.
   a. True
   b. False

9. Dorothy Grant stays in the relationship because she likes to be beaten and deliberately provokes the attacks on occasion.
   a. True
   b. False

Exercise 5

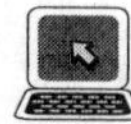

Virtual Hospital Activity

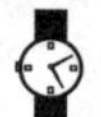

10 minutes

- Sign in to work at Pacific View Regional Hospital on the Obstetrics Floor for Period of Care 4. (*Note*: If you are already in the virtual hospital from a previous exercise, click on **Leave the Floor** and then on **Restart the Program** to get to the sign-in window.)
- From the Nurses' Station, click on **Kardex** and then on tab **201** to review Dorothy Grant's record. (*Remember:* You are not able to visit patients or administer medications during Period of Care 4. You are able to review patient records only.)

1. What action was initiated on Wednesday to protect Dorothy Grant from her husband?

Security will be notified if husband
comes to visit

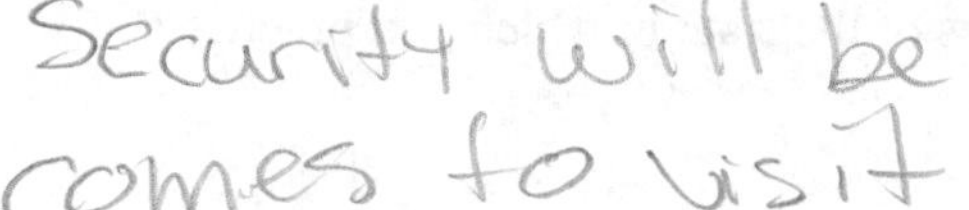

2. What nursing diagnoses are appropriate for this patient's current life situation?

3. What other disciplines have been contacted or consulted to ensure continuity of care for Dorothy Grant as it relates to her abuse?

- Social worker
- psychiatric team

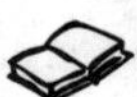 Review pages 570-573 in your textbook before answering the following questions.

4. As a nurse caring for Dorothy Grant, what is your responsibility for reporting IPV?

5. What are the reporting requirements of the state in which you practice?

6. What are the resources available in your area for women who are experiencing IPV?

LESSON 7

Pregnancy-Related Complications: Hemorrhagic Conditions of Late Pregnancy

Reading Assignment: Pregnancy-Related Complications (Chapter 25, pages 583-589)

Patient: Gabriela Valenzuela, Room 205

Goal: Demonstrate an understanding of the identification and management of selected hemorrhagic complications of pregnancy.

Objectives:

1. Identify appropriate interventions for managing abruptio placentae.
2. Differentiate between the symptoms related to an abruptio placentae and those related to a placenta previa.
3. Plan and evaluate essential patient education during the acute phase of diagnosis.

Exercise 1

Virtual Hospital Activity

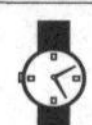

45 minutes

- Sign in to work at Pacific View Regional Hospital on the Obstetrics Floor for Period of Care 1. (*Note*: If you are already in the virtual hospital from a previous exercise, click on **Leave the Floor** and then on **Restart the Program** to get to the sign-in window.)
- From the Patient List, select Gabriela Valenzuela.
- Click on **Go to Nurses' Station**.
- Click on **Chart** and then on **205**.
- Click on **Emergency Department**.

1. What happened that precipitated Gabriela Valenzuela coming to the Emergency Department? How long did she wait before actually coming? What was the deciding factor in her coming to the Emergency Department?

Gabriela was in a car accident earlier in the day she came to the ER because of bright red vaginal bleeding approximately 100ml

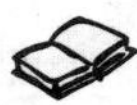 Read about the incidence and etiology of abruptio placentae in your textbook on page 585.

2. Other than a motor vehicle accident, what could result in or increase the risk for having an abruptio placentae?

- hypertension
- smoking
- multigravida status
- abdominal trauma from domestic violence
- history of previous premature separation of the placenta

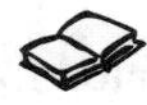 3. Differential diagnosis is very important when you are confronted with clinical manifestations that could be evidence of more than one process. Based on the information on pages 583-586 in your textbook, compare and contrast abruptio placentae and placenta previa in the table below and on the next page.

Characteristic/Complication	Abruptio Placentae	Placenta Previa
Bleeding	-sudden onset of painless uterine bleeding in the later half of pregnancy	- vaginal bleeding
Shock complication		- hypovolemic shock
Coagulopathy (DIC)		- Clotting abnormalities can be a danger to the woman

Characteristic/Complication	Abruptio Placentae	Placenta Previa
Uterine tonicity	- firm to stony hard	- High uterine resting tne
Tenderness/pain	- may have pain if active labor contractions are happening	- abdominal & low back pain described as aching or dull - Uterine tenderness that may be localized to site of abruption
Placenta findings - Total: Placenta completely covers internal cervical os	- Marginal: Placenta is implanted in the lower uterus but lower border is more than 3cm from internal cervical os - Partial: lower border is within 3cm of the internal cervical os but doest completly cover	
Fetal effects	- more likely to occure if fetus is male - fetus may be born early	- danger to the fetus related to anoxia, blood loss, and preterm birth

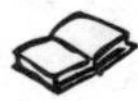

4. Based on your review of the Emergency Department report in the chart, what type of abruption does Gabriela Valenzuela have? Provide supporting documentation from your textbook reading. (*Hint*: Review Figure 25-5 on page 586 in your textbook.)

Gabriela has abruptio placentae becase She has vaginal bleeding, and abdominal pain

- Click on **Return to Nurses' Station**.
- Click on **205** to go to the patient's room.
- Click on the **Patient Care** and then on **Nurse-Client Interactions**.
- Select and view the video titled **0740: Patient Teaching—Fetal Monitoring**. (*Note*: Check the virtual clock to see whether enough time has elapsed. You can use the fast-forward feature to advance the time by 2-minute intervals if the video is not yet available. Then click again on **Patient Care** and **Nurse-Client Interactions** to refresh the screen.)

5. Once Gabriela Valenzuela is admitted to the floor, what are her and her husband's concerns? What does the nurse include in her teaching to alleviate those concerns?

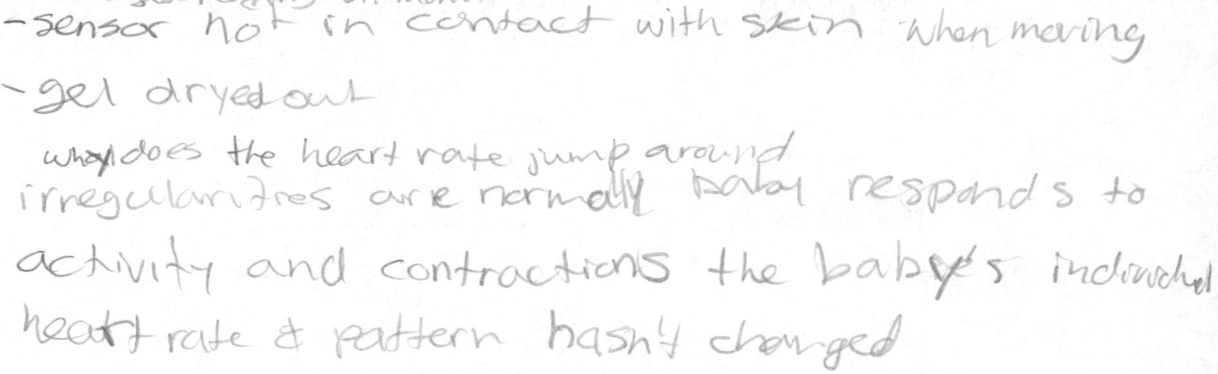

Gabriela Valenzuela is at increased risk for early delivery as a result of the abdominal trauma she suffered and the subsequent occurrence of a grade 1 abruptio placentae. She is currently manifesting signs and symptoms of early labor. According to the Physician's Orders, she was given a dose of betamethasone, which is to be repeated in 12 hours.

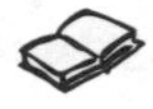

6. What is the purpose of the administration of betamethasone in this patient's case? (*Hint*: Review information on page 653 in your textbook.)

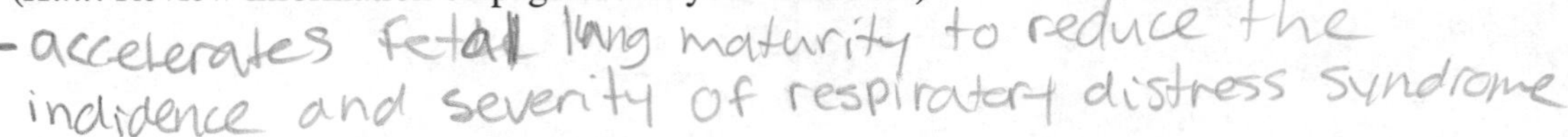

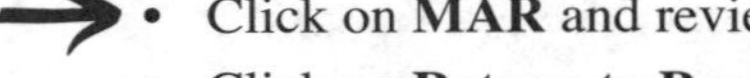

- Click on **MAR** and review the betamethasone dosage to be given to Gabriela Valenzuela.
- Click on **Return to Room 205**.
- Click on **Medication Room**.
- Click on **Unit Dosage**.
- Click on drawer **205**.
- Click on **Betamethasone** in the upper left corner of the screen.
- Click on **Put Medication on Tray**.
- Click on **Close Drawer**.
- Click on **View Medication Room**.
- Click on **Preparation**.
- Click on **Prepare** and follow the Preparation Wizard's prompts to complete preparation of Gabriela Valenzuela's betamethasone.
- When the Wizard stops asking questions, click on **Finish**.
- Click on **Return to Medication Room**.
- Click on **205** to return to the patient's room.
- Click on **Patient Care**.
- Click on **Medication Administration**.
- Click on **Review Your Medications**.
- Click on the tab marked **Prepared**.

7. According to the text box on the right side of your screen, what is the medication name and dosage that you have prepared for Gabriela Valenzuela?

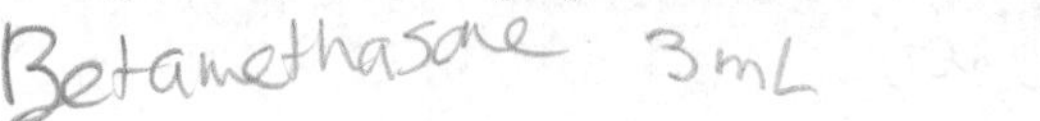

8. Based on your answer to the previous question, how many milligrams are you giving to Gabriela Valenzuela? Is this the correct dosage based on the MAR?

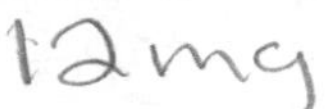

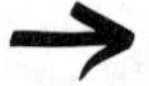

- Click on **Return to Room 205**.
- Click on the **Drug** icon in the left-hand corner of the screen.
- To read about betamethasone, either type the drug name in the search box or scroll through the alphabetic list of medications at the top of the screen.

9. Based on the information provided in the Drug Guide, what is the indication and dosage for pregnant adults?

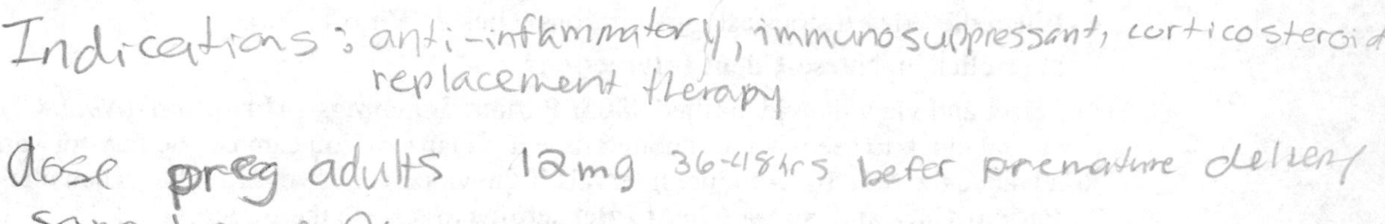

10. Based on your review of the baseline assessment data in the Drug Guide, what areas need to be assessed in Gabriela Valenzuela's history?

11. Now review the information regarding the administration of this medication. What are three things that need to be taken into consideration when giving this medication in the injection form?

- Avoide SC administration may damage tissue
- Inject deeply in large muscle mass avoid deltoid
- Use 21G needle
- Give in AM to prevent adrenal suppression

12. What are the six rights of medication administration as they relate to the patient?

Right medication
Right route
Right time
Right client
Right dose
Right documentation

You are now ready to complete the medication administration.

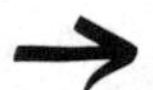

- Click on **Return to Room 205**.
- Click on **Check Armband**.
- Within the purple box under the patient's photo, find Betamethasone. Click the down arrow next to **Select** and choose **Administer**.
- Follow the Medication Wizard's prompts to administer Gabriela Valenzuela's betamethasone. Select **Yes** when asked whether to document the injection in the MAR.
- When the Wizard stops asking questions, click on **Finish**.
- Now click on **Nurse-Client Interactions**.
- Select and view the video titled **0805: Patient Teaching—Abruption**. (*Note*: Check the virtual clock to see whether enough time has elapsed. You can use the fast-forward feature to advance the time by 2-minute intervals if the video is not yet available. Then click again on **Patient Care** and **Nurse-Client Interactions** to refresh the screen.)

13. According to the video, what will help increase the oxygen supply to the baby and prevent further separation of the placenta?

→ prevent separation
Strick bed rest and laying on side can ↑ O_2 supply to baby because ↓ pressure on vessils that supplies O_2 to ~~baby~~ placental

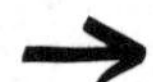

- Click on **Leave the Floor**.
- Click on **Look at Your Preceptor's Evaluation**.
- Click on **Medication Scorecard** and review the evaluation. How did you do? (*Hint:* For a quick refresher on reading your Medication Scorecard, see page 22 in the **Getting Started** section of this workbook. For a more detailed tour on preparing and administering medications and interpreting your Scorecard, see pages 26-30 and 37-41.)

Exercise 2

Virtual Hospital Activity

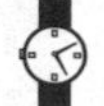

30 minutes

- Sign in to work at Pacific View Regional Hospital on the Obstetrics Floor for Period of Care 2. (*Note*: If you are already in the virtual hospital from a previous exercise, click on **Leave the Floor** and then on **Restart the Program** to get to the sign-in window.)
- From the Patient List, select Gabriela Valenzuela.
- Click on **Go to Nurses' Station**.
- Click on **Chart** and then on **205**.
- Click on **Diagnostic Reports**.

1. Gabriela Valenzuela had an ultrasound done on Tuesday to determine the source of the bleeding. What were the findings on the ultrasound?

- fetus in vertex presentation
- lowlying placenta with partial marginal abruption
- 3x3 clot noted

- Click on the **Laboratory Reports**.

2. What were Gabriela Valenzuela's hemoglobin and hematocrit levels on Tuesday? How do these findings compare with Wednesday's report? Has there been a significant change?

Tues hemo: 10.8 wed: 10.4
Tues hema: 34.1 wed: 32.4

3. According to the textbook information, it is important that the patient's hematocrit level be maintained above 33% . (*Hint:* See pages 291-292 in your textbook.)

Review page 586 in your textbook.

4. What clinical manifestations would indicate a worsening in the condition of either the patient or the fetus?

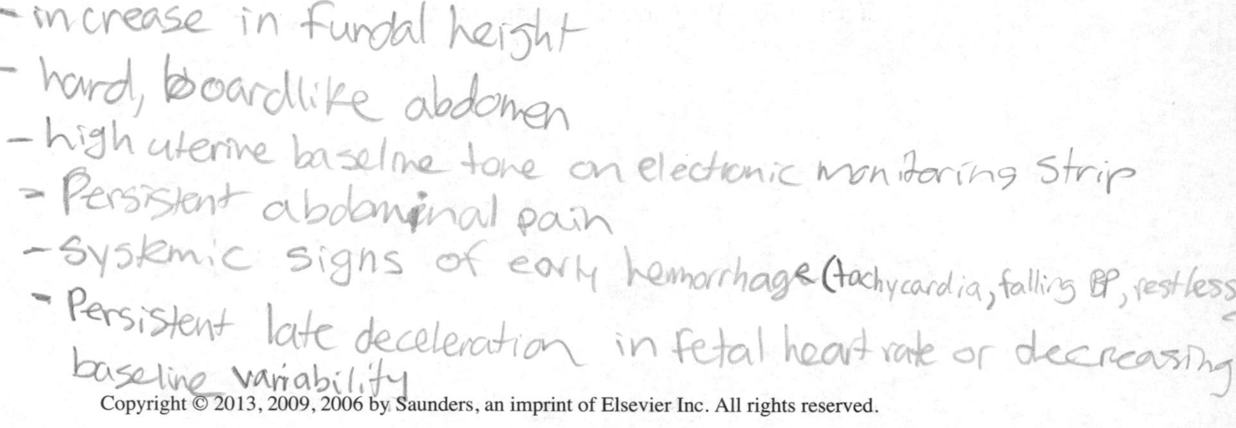

- Click on **Return to Nurses' Station**.
- Click on **EPR** and **Login**.
- Select **205** from the Patient drop-down menu and **Vital Signs** from the Category drop-down menu.
- Using the blue arrows, scroll to review the vital signs data over the last 12 hours.

5. From 0000 Wednesday until 1200 Wednesday, would you consider Gabriela Valenzuela's condition stable or unstable? State the rationale for your answer.

Pain: 3-4, 1, 1-2, 3-4
Temp: 97.8, 97.6, 98.2, 98.4
BP: 130/68, 126/66, 126/68, 126/70
H: 86, 72, 70, 86
R: 24, 18, 18, 18

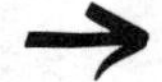

- Click on **Exit EPR**
- Click on **205** at the bottom of the screen.
- Click on **Patient Care** and then on **Nurse-Client Interactions**.
- Select and view the video titled **1140: Intervention—Bleeding, Comfort**. Take notes as you watch and listen. (*Note*: Check the virtual clock to see whether enough time has elapsed. You can use the fast-forward feature to advance the time by 2-minute intervals if the video is not yet available. Then click again on **Patient Care** and **Nurse-Client Interactions** to refresh the screen.)

6. What happened to elicit this interaction? (*Hint*: Review the Nurse's Notes for Wednesday 1140.)

Gush of about 50mL dark blood with clots when she got up to void. Complaint of increased pain (4-5/10) with contractions

7. What actions did the nurse take during the video?

- Reassured the patient and husband
- Told the patient she would inform the doctor
- Involved the husband to help with breathing technique

Exercise 3

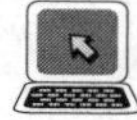

Virtual Hospital Activity

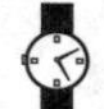

15 minutes

- Sign in to work at Pacific View Regional Hospital on the Obstetrics Floor for Period of Care 3. (*Note*: If you are already in the virtual hospital from a previous exercise, click on **Leave the Floor** and then on **Restart the Program** to get to the sign-in window.)
- From the Patient List, select Gabriela Valenzuela.
- Click on **Go to Nurses' Station**.
- Click on **Kardex** and then on tab **205**.

1. What problem areas have been identified by the nurse related to Gabriela Valenzuela's diagnosis?

Knowledge deficit: labor process, pain control

Comfort and pain

Hematology

2. What is the focus of the desired outcomes related to the problems you listed in question 1?

Patient will understand labor process, pain control

Patient will have reduced or minimal pain

Patient/family will achieve understanding of their disease process

3. Using correct NANDA nursing diagnosis terminology, write four possible nursing diagnoses appropriate for Gabriela Valenzuela at this time.

- Risk for acute pain related to uterine contractions
- Anxiety related to unknown outcome and change in birth plans
- Risk for ineffective health maintenance related to deficient knowledge regarding self-care with disorder
- Risk for deficient fluid volume related to hemorrhage

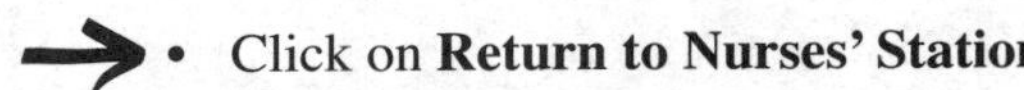

- Click on **Return to Nurses' Station**.
- Click on **Chart**.
- Click on **205**.
- Click on **Patient Education**.

4. According to the Patient Education sheet in Gabriela Valenzuela's chart, what are the educational goals related to the patient's diagnosis?

- Understand preterm infant and need for NICU care
- State the benefits of breast feeding a preterm infant
- Understand labor process including monitoring & medication
- Understanding of abruption protocol & ultrasound results

- Click on **Nurse's Notes**.

5. What education has been completed by the nurses through Period of Care 3? Include the times and topics discussed.

6. What are some barriers to learning that the nurse may confront with this patient?

7. How can the nurse overcome each of the barriers you identified in the previous question?

LESSON 8

Pregnancy-Related Complications: Hypertension During Pregnancy

Reading Assignment: Pregnancy-Related Complications (Chapter 25, pages 590-601)

Patient: Kelly Brady, Room 203

Goal: Demonstrate an understanding of the identification and management of severe preeclampsia.

Objectives:

1. Assess and identify signs and symptoms present in the patient with severe preeclampsia.
2. Explain how common signs and symptoms present in the patient with severe preeclampsia relate to the underlying pathophysiology of this disease.
3. Identify the patient who has developed HELLP syndrome.
4. Describe routine nursing care for the patient with severe preeclampsia who is receiving magnesium sulfate.

Exercise 1

Virtual Hospital Activity

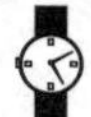

20 minutes

- Sign in to work at Pacific View Regional Hospital on the Obstetrics Floor for Period of Care 3. (*Note*: If you are already in the virtual hospital from a previous exercise, click on **Leave the Floor** and then on **Restart the Program** to get to the sign-in window.)
- From the Patient List, select Kelly Brady.
- Click on **Go to Nurses' Station**.
- Click on **Chart** and then on **203**.
- Click on **History and Physical**.

Hemolysis
Elevated
Liver enzymes
Low
Platelets

1. What was Kelly Brady's admission diagnosis?

probable severe preeclampsia

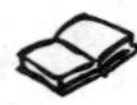

2. Using Kelly Brady's History and Physical, as well as Table 25-3 on page 594 in your textbook, complete the table below.

Sign/Symptom	Mild Preeclampsia	Severe Preeclampsia	Kelly Brady on Admission
Blood pressure Systolic BP	≥140 but <160mm Hg	≥160mm Hg 2 readings 6hrs apart while on bed rest	183/~~100~~
Diastolic BP	≥90 but <110mm Hg	≥110mm Hg	100
Proteinuria 24hr specimen preferred to eliminate hr to hr variation	≥0.3g but <2g in 24hr specimen (1+ or higher on random dipstick)	≥5g in 24hr specimen (3+ higher on random dipstick samples)	4660mg
Headache (severe, unrelenting, not attributable to other cause)	absent	often present	complaint of headach x2days acetaminophen doesnt help
Visual disturbances (spots or "sparkles"; temporary blindness; photophobia)	absent to minimal	common	no blurred vision
Right upper quadrant or epigastric pain	absent	may be present & often precedes seizure	no complaint

- Click on **Physician's Orders** and find the admitting physician's orders on Tuesday at 1030.

3. What tests and/or procedures did Kelly Brady's physician order to confirm the diagnosis of severe preeclampsia?

- 24 hr urine for total protein
- vitals q4h notifiy MD of diastolic BPs >110

- Click on **Physician's Notes** and scroll to the note for Wednesday 0730.

4. What subjective and objective data are recorded here that would support the diagnosis of severe preeclampsia?

- severe headache
- BPs overnight 163-192/90-102

Kelly Brady's 24-hour urine collection was completed and sent to the lab at 1230.

- Click on **Laboratory Reports**.
- Scroll to find the Wednesday 1230 results.

5. Below, record the results of Kelly Brady's 24-hour urine collection.

Total volume 2000
Protein 4660 mg
creatinine 110.3
" clearance 255.3

Exercise 2

Virtual Hospital Activity

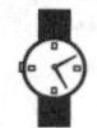

20 minutes

- Sign in to work at Pacific View Regional Hospital on the Obstetrics Floor for Period of Care 1. (*Note*: If you are already in the virtual hospital from a previous exercise, click on **Leave the Floor** and then on **Restart the Program** to get to the sign-in window.)
- From the Patient List, select Kelly Brady.
- Click on **Go to Nurses' Station**.
- Click on **203** at the bottom of the screen to go to the patient's room.
- Click on **Take Vital Signs**.

1. Below, record Kelly Brady's vital signs for 0730.

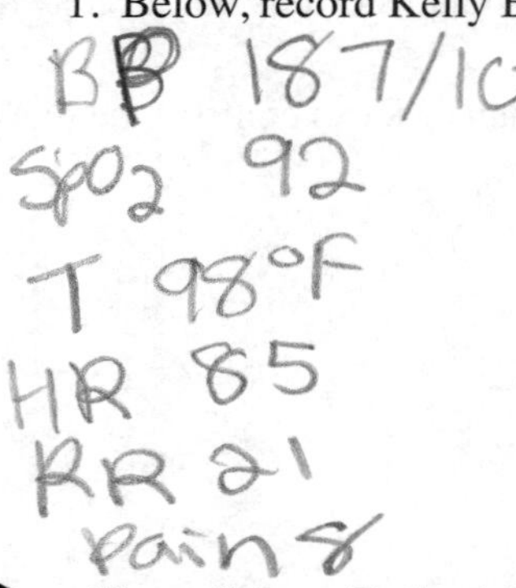

- Now click on **Patient Care**. To perform a focused assessment, select the various body system categories (yellow buttons) and subcategories (green buttons) as listed in question 2.

2. Record your findings from the focused assessment of Kelly Brady in the table below.

Assessment Area	Kelly Brady's Findings
Head and Neck Sensory	-pupils bilaterally equal & reactive to light -denies blurred vision, discharge, or cerumen -nares clear without redness, swelling, or discharge
Neurologic	-cranial nerves intact without apparent deficits -complains of continuous occipital headache for 2 days which is worse with physical activity. reports pain 8/10
Chest Respiratory	-resp effort regular & even -bilateral breathsounds clear & equal to auscultation -no adventitious lung sounds -mildly tachypneic with pain 8/10 -no cough -no accessory muscles -SpO_2 92% RA
Abdomen Gastrointestinal	-Bowel sounds ausclutaten in all 4 quadrants -no palpable tenderness or masses -denies epigastric or right upper quadrant abdominal pain
Lower Extremities Neurologic	-no tremors or weakness -reflexes intact -deep tendon reflexes (DTR) 2+ without clonus -sensation intact

3. Preeclampsia is a result of hypertension resulting in an overall decreased blood flow to organs.

4. Match each of the signs or symptoms below with the preeclampsia-associated pathology it indicates. (*Note:* Some letters will be used more than once.)

	Sign or Symptom	**Pathology**
c	Blurred vision/blind spots	a. Generalized vasoconstriction
c	Headache	b. Glomerular damage
d	Epigastric pain	c. Vasoconstriction of cerebral vessels; arterial vasospasm
c	Hyperreflexia	d. Hepatic edema and subcapsular hemorrhage; hemorrhagic necrosis
a	Elevated blood pressure	
b	Proteinuria/oliguria	

Exercise 3

Virtual Hospital Activity

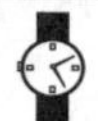

30 minutes

- Sign in to work at Pacific View Regional Hospital on the Obstetrics Floor for Period of Care 3. (*Note*: If you are already in the virtual hospital from a previous exercise, click on **Leave the Floor** and then on **Restart the Program** to get to the sign-in window.)
- From the Patient List, select Kelly Brady.
- Click on **Go to Nurses' Station**.

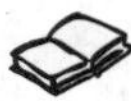

Read about HELLP syndrome on pages 600-601 in your textbook.

1. Why do you think Kelly Brady had blood drawn at 1230 for an AST measurement and a platelet count?

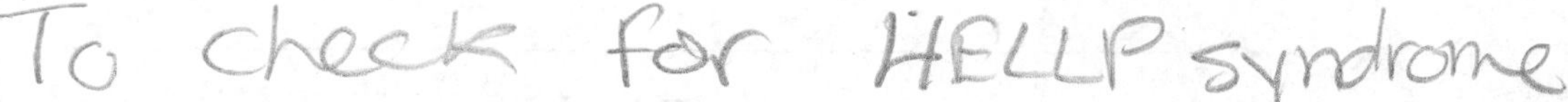

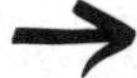

- Click on **Chart** and then on **203**.
- Click on **Laboratory Reports**.
- Scroll to the report for Wednesday 1230 to locate the results of these tests.

2. Complete the table below based on your review of the Laboratory Reports and your textbook.

Test	Wed 1230 Result	Value in HELLP
Platelet count	55 000	
AST Aspartate aminotransferase	184	

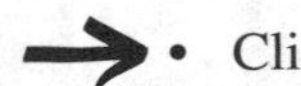

- Click on **Return to Nurses' Station**.
- Click on **Patient List** (on the tool bar at the top of the screen).
- Click on **Get Report** for Kelly Brady.

3. Why has Kelly Brady been transferred to labor and delivery?

becase she was diagnosed with HELLP syndrome

4. HELLP syndrome consists of intravascular damage, increase liver enzymes, and low platelet count.

The prominent symptom of HELLP syndrome is pain in the right upper quadrent, the lower chest, or epigastric area.

Other signs and symptoms include nausea, vomiting, and severe edema

- Click on **Return to Patient List** and then on **Return to Nurses' Station.**
- Click on **Chart** and then on **203**.
- Click on **Physician's Notes**.
- Scroll to the note for Wednesday 1530.

5. What is the physician's plan of care for Kelly Brady, in light of the HELLP syndrome diagnosis?

immediate delivery by cesarean section at 2000. Magnesium sulfate for 24 hours after surgery for seizure prophylaxis

Assume that you will be the nurse caring for Kelly Brady after her surgery while she is receiving magnesium sulfate. Read about this medication on pages 594-597 in your textbook and then answer question 6.

6. All of the assessments/interventions listed below are part of routine nursing care for a patient with severe preeclampsia. Which of these are performed specifically to assess for magnesium toxicity? Select all that apply.

✓ Measure/record urine output.

_____ Measure proteinuria using urine dipstick.

_____ Monitor liver enzyme levels and platelet count.

_____ Monitor for headache, visual disturbances, and epigastric pain.

✓ Assess for decreased level of consciousness.

✓ Assess DTRs.

_____ Weigh daily to assess for edema.

✓ Monitor vital signs, especially respiratory rate.

_____ Dim room lights and maintain a quiet environment.

LESSON **9**

Concurrent Disorders During Pregnancy: Gestational Diabetes Mellitus

Reading Assignment: Concurrent Disorders During Pregnancy (Chapter 26, pages 607-616)

Patient: Stacey Crider, Room 202

Goal: Demonstrate an understanding of the identification and management of gestational diabetes mellitus (GDM).

Objectives:

1. Identify appropriate interventions for controlling hyperglycemia in a patient with GDM.
2. Correctly administer insulin to a patient with GDM.
3. Plan and evaluate essential patient teaching for a patient with GDM.

Exercise 1

Virtual Hospital Activity

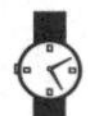

30 minutes

- Sign in to work at Pacific View Regional Hospital on the Obstetrics Floor for Period of Care 2. (*Note*: If you are already in the virtual hospital from a previous exercise, click on **Leave the Floor** and then on **Restart the Program** to get to the sign-in window.)
- From the Patient List, select Stacey Crider.
- Click on **Go to Nurses' Station**.
- Click on **Chart** and then on **202**.
- Click on **History and Physical**.

1. When was Stacey Crider's GDM diagnosed? How has it been managed so far?

- DX in first trimester
- unresponsive to diet by end of 1st trimester, began insulin with improved glycemic control, but not optimal

2. Read about risk factors for GDM on page 613 in your textbook. List these factors below.

- overweight (BMI 25-29.9 kg/m²), obese (BMI 30-39.9kg/m²), or morbidly obese (BMI ≥ 40kg/m²)
- Maternal age older than 25yrs
- GDM in previous pregnancy
- history of abnormal glucose tolerance
- history of diabetes in a close relative
- Member of a high-risk ethnic group (Hispanic, African, Native american, south or east Asian, or Pacific Islans ancestry)

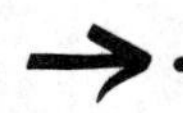

- To search for evidence of the above risk factors in Stacey Crider, continue reviewing her History and Physical and then click on and review her **Nursing Admission**.

3. Which risk factors for GDM are present in Stacey Crider?

- obesity BMI 34
- both parents and brother type 2 diabetic, Sister had GDM

4. What does Stacey Crider's physician suspect is the cause of her poorly controlled blood glucose levels? (*Hint*: See the Impression section at the end of her History and Physical.)

- PTL
- Bacterial vaginosis
- Poorly controlled gestational diabetes (noncompliance with diet)

- Click on **Physician's Orders**.

5. Look at Stacey Crider's admission orders. Write down the orders that are related to GDM.

Change Insulin Lispro to use premeal algorithm
Breakfast: if premeal glucos is: <60: Give 18 units
61-80: Give 19 units
81-100: Give 20 units

6. Why did Stacey Crider's physician order an HbA_{1C} test as part of her admission labs? (*Hint*: See page 611 in your textbook.)

The HbA1c test was ordered to check Stacey's glycosylated hemoglobin. This test is used because it's not affected by recent intake or restriction of food, therefore it can detect prolonged hyperglycemia

On admission, Stacey Crider was in preterm labor. This was treated with magnesium sulfate tocolysis. She was also given a course of betamethasone.

- Click on **Return to Nurses' Station**.
- Click on the **Drug** icon in the lower left corner of the screen.
- Use the search box or scroll bar to find the entry for betamethasone.

7. How might betamethasone affect Stacey Crider's GDM?

Betamethasone can increase blood glucose levels

- Click on **Return to Nurses' Station**.
- Click on **Chart** and then on **202**.
- Click on **Physician's Notes**.
- Scroll to the note for Tuesday at 0700.

8. How does Stacey Crider's physician plan to deal with these potential medication effects?

Double insulin doses while on betamethasone

Stacey Crider's other admission diagnosis is bacterial vaginosis (BV).

- Click on **Return to Nurses' Station**.
- Click on **202** at the bottom of your screen.
- Click on **Patient Care** and then on **Nurse-Client Interactions**.
- Select and view the video titled **1115: Teaching—Diet, Infection**. (*Note*: Check the virtual clock to see whether enough time has elapsed. You can use the fast-forward feature to advance the time by 2-minute intervals if the video is not yet available. Then click again on **Patient Care** and **Nurse-Client Interactions** to refresh the screen.)

9. What is the relationship between Stacey Crider's bacterial vaginosis infection and her GDM? (increased bacterial growth in nutrient-rich urine p613)

Stacey's blood sugars are high so it ~~puts her at an~~ makes her more suseptible to infections

high glucos favorable envirment for bacteria

Exercise 2

Virtual Hospital Activity

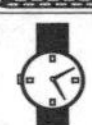

20 minutes

- Sign in to work at Pacific View Regional Hospital on the Obstetrics Floor for Period of Care 1. (*Note*: If you are already in the virtual hospital from a previous exercise, click on **Leave the Floor** and then on **Restart the Program** to get to the sign-in window.)
- From the Patient List, select Stacey Crider.
- Click on **Go to Nurses' Station**.
- Click on the **Drug** icon in the lower left corner.

Stacey Crider needs her insulin so that she can eat breakfast. Remember that she receives lispro insulin prior to each meal and NPH insulin at bedtime. Read about the different types of insulin in the Drug Guide.

1. Using the information found in the Pharmacokinetics section of the entry for insulin in the Drug Guide, complete the table below.

Type of Insulin	Onset of Action	Peak	Duration
Lispro	¼ hr	½ - 1½ hr	4-5 hrs
NPH	1-2 hr	6-14 h	24+ hrs

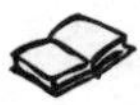 Read about proper insulin injection technique in your textbook on page 643.

- Click on **EPR** and then on **Login**.
- Select **202** from the Patient drop-down menu and **Vital Signs** from the Category drop-down menu.
- Look at the vital sign assessment documented on Wednesday at 0700.

2. What was Stacey Crider's blood glucose?

110

- Click on **Exit EPR**.
- Click on **MAR**.
- Click on tab **202**.

3. What is Stacey Crider's prescribed insulin dosage?

22 units

- Click on **Return to Nurses' Station**.
- Click on **Chart** and then on **202**.
- Click on **Physician's Orders** and scroll to the orders for Tuesday at 1900.

4. How much insulin should Stacey Crider receive? Why?

At breakfast she gets 22unit when her sugar isbetween 101-130

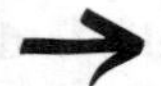

- Click on **Return to Nurses' Station**.
- Click on **Medication Room**.
- Click on **Unit Dosage**.
- Click on drawer **202**.
- Click on **Insulin Lispro**.
- Click on **Put Medication on Tray**.
- Click on **Close Drawer**.
- Click on **View Medication Room**.
- Click on **Preparation**.
- Click on **Prepare** and follow the prompts to complete preparation of Stacey Crider's lispro insulin dose.
- Click on **Return to Medication Room**.

You are almost ready to give Stacey Crider's insulin injection. However, before you do . . .

5. Considering lispro insulin's rapid onset of action, what else should you check before giving Stacey Crider her injection?

Now you're ready!

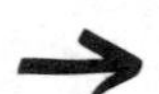

- Click on Room **202**.
- Click on **Check Armband**.
- Click on **Patient Care**.
- Click on **Medication Administration**.
- Insulin Lispro should be listed on the left side of your screen. Click on the down arrow next to **Select** and choose **Administer**.
- Follow the prompts to administer Stacey Crider's insulin injection. Indicate **Yes** to document the injection in the MAR.
- Click on **Leave the Floor**.
- Click on **Look at Your Preceptor's Evaluation**.
- Click on **Medication Scorecard**. How did you do?

Exercise 3

Virtual Hospital Activity

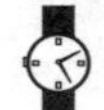

30 minutes

- Sign in to work at Pacific View Regional Hospital on the Obstetrics Floor for Period of Care 3. (*Note*: If you are already in the virtual hospital from a previous exercise, click on **Leave the Floor** and then on **Restart the Program** to get to the sign-in window.)
- From the Patient List, select Stacey Crider.
- Click on **Go to Nurses' Station**.
- Click on **Chart** and then on **202**.
- Click on **Patient Education**.

Stacey Crider will likely be discharged home soon. Review her Patient Education record to determine her learning needs in relation to GDM.

1. List the educational goals for Stacey Crider regarding GDM.

- verbalize appropriate food choices and portions
- Demonstrate good technique when administering insulin
- Demonstrate good technique with self-monitoring blood glucose
- recognize hyper and hypoglycemia and how to treat each

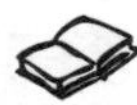

Read Nursing Care: The Pregnant Woman with Diabetes Mellitus on pages 614-616 in your textbook.

2. Which of Stacey Crider's educational goals would *not* apply to all women with GDM? Support your answer.

➔ • Click on **Nurse's Notes** and scroll to the note for 0600 Wednesday.

3. How did the nurse describe Stacey Crider's ability to give her own insulin injection at that time?

Gives injection in her arm instead of abdomen. Seems uncertain when reading units on syringe

➔ • Click again on **Patient Education**.

4. What teaching has already been done with this patient on Wednesday in regard to GDM?

She has been taught about: food choices, insulin administration, SMBG, S&S of hyper/hypoglycemia.

➔ • Click on **Nurse's Notes** and scroll to the note for 1200 Wednesday.

5. Do you think today's initial teaching on insulin administration was effective? Support your answer using objective documentation from the Nurse's Note.

Yes because the patient stated "I am feeling better about giving myself insulin.

Use the information you have obtained from the Patient Education form and the Nurse's Notes to answer the following questions.

6. Teaching goals for Stacey Crider include all of the following. Which goal(s) would you choose to work on with her during *this* period of care? Select all that apply.

✓ Verbalize appropriate food choices and portions.

✓ Demonstrate good technique when administering insulin.

_____ Demonstrate good technique with self-monitoring of blood glucose.

_____ Recognize hyper- and hypoglycemia and how to treat each.

7. Give a rationale for your answer to question 6.

Pt stated she needs to work on sticking to the diet better.

8. Which goal do you think Stacey Crider would choose to work on during this period of care?

✓ Verbalize appropriate food choices and portions.

_____ Demonstrate good technique when administering insulin.

_____ Demonstrate good technique with self-monitoring of blood glucose.

_____ Recognize hyper- and hypoglycemia and how to treat each.

9. Give a rationale for your answer to question 8.

based on the pt education sheet she still requires some supervision

Read Risk Factors for Gestational Diabetes Mellitus on page 613 in your textbook.

10. Stacey Crider has a significant risk for developing glucose intolerance later in life. What advice would you give her to reduce this risk?

I would advice Stacey to stick with her diet ~~and~~ to help control her sugar levels and help her loose weight which will help reduce her risk of developing glucose intolerance.

11. Because she has had GDM with this pregnancy, what medical follow-up would you advise for Stacey Crider after her baby is born? Why?

After birt Blood glucose levels should be monitered at least 4 x daily, so insulin dose can be adjusted.

Postpartum Screening at 6-12 weeks is recommended to identify diabetes or impaired glucose metabolism. and determin if any intervention is needed

12. Do you believe Stacey Crider's GDM might affect her child? What advice would you give her regarding medical follow-up for her baby?

LESSON 10

Concurrent Disorders During Pregnancy: Cardiac Disease/Anemia/Lupus

Reading Assignment: Concurrent Disorders During Pregnancy (Chapter 26, pages 616-624)

Patients: Maggie Gardner, Room 204
Gabriela Valenzuela, Room 205

Goal: Demonstrate an understanding of the identification and management of selected medical-surgical problems in pregnancy.

Objectives:

1. Identify appropriate interventions for managing selected medical-surgical problems in pregnancy.
2. Plan and evaluate essential patient education during the acute phase of diagnosis.

Exercise 1

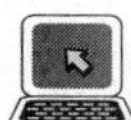

Virtual Hospital Activity

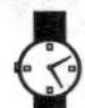

10 minutes

- Sign in to work at Pacific View Regional Hospital on the Obstetrics Floor for Period of Care 1. (*Note*: If you are already in the virtual hospital from a previous exercise, click on **Leave the Floor** and then on **Restart the Program** to get to the sign-in window.)
- From the Patient List, select Gabriela Valenzuela.
- Click on **Go to Nurses' Station**.
- Click on **Chart** and then on **205**.
- Click on **History and Physical**.

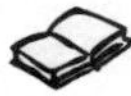

Review material regarding cardiac problems during pregnancy on pages 616-621 in your textbook.

1. In the History and Physical for Gabriela Valenzuela, what does the physician note as her cardiac problem?

2. Mitral valve disease is one of the most common causes of cardiac disease in pregnant women.
   a. True
   b. False

3. According to the History and Physical, what cardiac symptoms does Gabriela Valenzuela exhibit now that she is pregnant?

4. Based on your textbook reading, why do pregnant women with cardiac disorders have problems during their pregnancy?

5. What abnormal assessment finding is noted in the History and Physical that would be associated with Gabriela Valenzuela's cardiac disorder?

Exercise 2

Virtual Hospital Activity

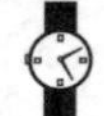

20 minutes

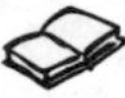

Autoimmune disorders encompass a wide variety of disorders that can be disruptive to the pregnancy process. Maggie Gardner has been admitted to rule out systemic lupus erythematosus (SLE). The following activities will explore the various aspects of this autoimmune disorder. Review the information regarding SLE on page 623 in your textbook.

- Sign in to work at Pacific View Regional Hospital on the Obstetrics Floor for Period of Care 1. (*Note*: If you are already in the virtual hospital from a previous exercise, click on **Leave the Floor** and then on **Restart the Program** to get to the sign-in window.)
- From the Patient List, select Maggie Gardner.
- Click on **Go to Nurses' Station**.
- Click on **Chart** and then on **204**.
- Click on **History and Physical**.

1. Based on Maggie Gardner's History and Physical, what information would correlate to a diagnosis of SLE?

2. According to the textbook, what are most often the presenting symptom of this disease during pregnancy?

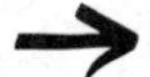

- Click on **Return to Nurses' Station**.
- Click on **204** at the bottom of the screen.
- Click on **Patient Care** and then on **Physical Assessment**.
- Click on the various body system categories (yellow buttons) and subcategories (green buttons) to perform a head-to-toe assessment of Maggie Gardner.

3. Based on your head-to-toe assessment, list four abnormal findings that are related to Maggie Gardner's diagnosis.

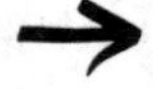

- Click on **Chart** and then on **204**.
- Click on **Patient Education**.

4. Based on your physical assessment, the information from the Patient Education section of the chart, and the fact that this is a new diagnosis for the patient, list three areas of teaching that need to be completed with this patient.

Exercise 3

Virtual Hospital Activity

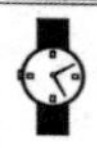

35 minutes

- Sign in to work at Pacific View Regional Hospital on the Obstetrics Floor for Period of Care 3. (*Note*: If you are already in the virtual hospital from a previous exercise, click on **Leave the Floor** and then on **Restart the Program** to get to the sign-in window.)
- From the Patient List, select Maggie Gardner.
- Click on **Go to Nurses' Station**.
- Click on **Chart** and then on **204**.
- Click on **Consultations** and review the Rheumatology Consult.

1. List four things noted in the rheumatologist's impressions regarding specific findings that are associated with a diagnosis of SLE for Maggie Gardner.

- Click on **Diagnostic Reports**.

2. Maggie Gardner had an ultrasound done before the consultation with the rheumatologist. What were the findings as they relate to SLE? What were the follow-up recommendations? (*Hint*: See Impressions section.)

3. What is the rheumatologist's plan regarding laboratory/diagnostics to gain a definitive diagnosis?

4. According to the Rheumatology Consult, what is the plan regarding medications (immediate need)?

- Click on **Return to Nurses' Station**.
- Click on the **Drug** icon in the lower left corner of the screen.
- Find the Drug Guide profile of prednisone. (*Hint:* You can type the drug name in the search box or scroll through the alphabetic list of drugs at the top of the screen.)

5. What does Maggie Gardner need to be taught regarding this medication?

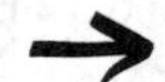

- Click on **Return to Nurses' Station**.
- Click on **204**.
- Click on **Patient Care** and then on **Nurse-Client Interactions**.
- Select and view the video titled **1530: Disease Management**. (*Note*: Check the virtual clock to see whether enough time has elapsed. You can use the fast-forward feature to advance the time by 2-minute intervals if the video is not yet available. Then click again on **Patient Care** and **Nurse-Client Interactions** to refresh the screen.)

6. During this video, the nurse provides Maggie Gardner with information regarding her disease. What two things does the nurse note that are important aspects of the patient's disease management during pregnancy?

7. What medication, ordered by the rheumatologist, will assist in the blood flow to the placenta? How?

8. What key component does the nurse identify for Maggie Gardner that will assist in maintaining a healthy pregnancy?

9. What excuse does Maggie Gardner provide for not keeping previous doctor's appointments? (*Hint:* This information is also found in the Nursing Admission in the chart.)

Exercise 4

Virtual Hospital Activity

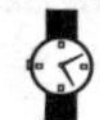

15 minutes

- Sign in to work at Pacific View Regional Hospital on the Obstetrics Floor for Period of Care 4. (*Note*: If you are already in the virtual hospital from a previous exercise, click on **Leave the Floor** and then on **Restart the Program** to get to the sign-in window.)
- From the Nurses' Station, click on **Chart**. (*Remember:* You are not able to visit patients or administer medications during Period of Care 4. You are able to review patient records only.)
- Click on **204** to open Maggie Gardner's chart.
- Click on **Laboratory Reports**.

1. The results are now available for the following laboratory tests that were ordered for Maggie Gardner during Period of Care 2. What are the findings?

Laboratory Test	Maggie Gardner's Result
C3	
C4	
CH50	
RPR	
ANA titer	
Anticardiolipin	
Anti-sm; Anti-DNA; Anti–SSA	
Anti-SSB	
Anti-RVV; Antiphospholipid	

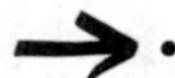• Click on **Consultations** and review the Rheumatology Consult.

2. The lab findings you recorded in question 1 are definitive for the diagnosis of SLE. According to the textbook and the Rheumatology Consult, what is the plan to manage this disease once Maggie Gardner's baby is delivered?

• Click on **Nurse's Notes.**

3. By Period of Care 4, Maggie Gardner has been provided with education regarding various aspects of her disease process, testing, and hospital procedures. Based on your review of the Nurse's Notes for Wednesday, what has she been specifically taught? Include the time each topic of instruction took place.

4. Using correct NANDA nursing diagnosis terminology, write three possible nursing diagnoses for Maggie Gardner.

5. SLE requires long-term management because patients will experience remissions and exacerbations. What step did the rheumatologist take with Maggie Gardner to begin the long-term relationship that will be required to ensure a healthy outcome?

LESSON 11

Concurrent Disorders During Pregnancy: Infections

Reading Assignment: Concurrent Disorders During Pregnancy (Chapter 26, pages 624-632)

Patients: Gabriela Valenzuela, Room 205
Laura Wilson, Room 206

Goal: Demonstrate an understanding of the identification and management of selected sexually transmitted infections and other infections in pregnant women.

Objectives:

1. Explain the importance of prophylactic Group B streptococcus (GBS) treatment.
2. Identify risk factors for acquiring the human immunodeficiency virus (HIV).
3. Prioritize information to be included in patient teaching related to HIV.

Exercise 1

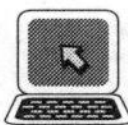

Virtual Hospital Activity

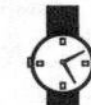

15 minutes

- Sign in to work at Pacific View Regional Hospital on the Obstetrics Floor for Period of Care 1. (*Note*: If you are already in the virtual hospital from a previous exercise, click on **Leave the Floor** and then on **Restart the Program** to get to the sign-in window.)
- From the Patient List, select Gabriela Valenzuela.
- Click on **Go to Nurses' Station**.
- Click on **Chart** and then on **205**.
- Click on **History and Physical** and scroll to the plan at the end of this document.

1. Is Gabriela Valenzuela known to be positive for GBS?

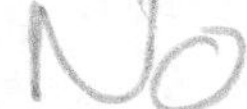

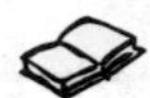 Read about GBS on pages 630-631 in your textbook; then answer questions 2 through 5.

2. List risk factors for neonatal GBS infection. Which risk factor applies to Gabriela Valenzuela?

Risk factors
- preterm labor *
- maternal intrapartum fever
- prolonged rupture of membranes
- previous birth of infected infant
- GBS bacteriuria in current pregnancy

3. Since pregnant women with GBS in the vagina are almost always asymptomatic, why does Gabriela Valenzuela need to be treated for this organism?

to prevent transmition of GBS to the infant.

- Click on **Physician's Orders**.
- Scroll to the admission orders written Tuesday at 2100.

4. What medication, dosage, and frequency will Gabriela Valenzuela receive for GBS prophylaxis?

- Betamethasone 12mg IM q12h 2 doses
- Ampicillin 2g IV q6h until dilivery

5. How does this order compare with the treatment regimen recommended in your textbook?

Normally it's ampicillin 2g initial dose IV followed by 1g IV q4h until childbirth

Exercise 2

Virtual Hospital Activity

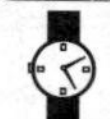

35 minutes

- Sign in to work at Pacific View Regional Hospital on the Obstetrics Floor for Period of Care 1. (*Note*: If you are already in the virtual hospital from a previous exercise, click on **Leave the Floor** and then on **Restart the Program** to get to the sign-in window.)
- From the Patient List, select Laura Wilson.
- Click on **Go to Nurses' Station**.
- Click on **Chart** and then on **206**.
- Click on **Nursing Admission**.

1. What risk factors for acquiring a sexually transmitted disease (STD) are identified on Laura Wilson's Nursing Admission form?

drug use
- multiple sex partners

2. In the United States, which group of women have the highest HIV infection rate?
   a. Black women
   b. White women
   c. Hispanic women

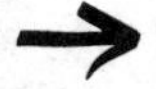

- While still in the chart, click on **Admissions**.

3. In the United States today, HIV infection is spreading most rapidly in the groups listed below. Identify the group(s) to which Laura Wilson belongs. Select all that apply.

✓ White women

_____ Black women

_____ Hispanic women

- Now click again on **Nursing Admission**.

4. What did the admitting nurse document about Laura Wilson's knowledge and acceptance of her HIV diagnosis?

Believes many people are positive and do just fine
Getting HIV was bad luck.
Believes taking ZDV will prevent AIDS & her baby has little to no risk of contracting virus

- Click on **Return to Nurses' Station** and then on **206** to visit the patient.
- Click on **Patient Care** and then on **Nurse-Client Interactions**.
- Select and view the video titled **0800: Teaching—HIV in Pregnancy**. (*Note*: Check the virtual clock to see whether enough time has elapsed. You can use the fast-forward feature to advance the time by 2-minute intervals if the video is not yet available. Then click again on **Patient Care** and **Nurse-Client Interactions** to refresh the screen.)

5. Does Laura Wilson appear to be fully aware of the implications of HIV infection? State the rationale for your answer.

No. She doesn't really seem to be fully aware. She seems to think that the risk of transmition is really low and that her baby won't get HIV

6. What coping mechanism is Laura Wilson exhibiting in the video interaction?

denial.

- Click on **Chart** and then on **206**.
- Click on **Nursing Admission**.

7. Laura Wilson needs education on all of the following topics. Which one would you choose to teach her about at this time?

_____ Safer sex

_____ Medication side effects and importance of compliance

_____ Need for medical follow-up and medication for the baby

__✓__ Impact of HIV on birth plans

8. Give a rationale for your answer to question 7.

It's important for Laura to know that changing her birth plans to having a csection can redue the risk of transmition of HIV to the baby

LESSON 12

The Woman with an Intrapartum Complication

Reading Assignment: Nursing Care During Obstetric Procedures (Chapter 19, pages 424-431)
The Woman with an Intrapartum Complication (Chapter 27)

Patients: Dorothy Grant, Room 201
Stacey Crider, Room 202
Kelly Brady, Room 203
Gabriela Valenzuela, Room 205

Goal: Demonstrate an understanding of the identification and management of selected labor and birth complications.

Objectives:

1. Assess and identify signs and symptoms present in the patient with preterm labor.
2. Describe appropriate nursing care for the patient in preterm labor.
3. Develop a birth plan to meet the needs of the preterm infant.

Exercise 1

Virtual Hospital Activity

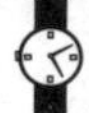

20 minutes

- Sign in to work at Pacific View Regional Hospital on the Obstetrics Floor for Period of Care 2. (*Note*: If you are already in the virtual hospital from a previous exercise, click on **Leave the Floor** and then on **Restart the Program** to get to the sign-in window.)
- From the Patient List, select Dorothy Grant and Gabriela Valenzuela.
- Click on **Go to Nurses' Station**.
- Click on **Chart** and then on **201** for Dorothy Grant's chart.
- Click on **History and Physical**.

1. Using the information found in the History and Physical section, complete the table below for Dorothy Grant.

Patient	Weeks Gestation	Reason for Admission
Dorothy Grant		

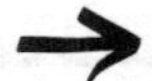

- Click on **Return to Nurses' Station**.
- Now click again on **Chart**; this time, select **205**.
- Click on **History and Physical**.

2. Using the information found in the History and Physical section, complete the table below for Gabriela Valenzuela.

Patient	Weeks Gestation	Reason for Admission
Gabriela Valenzuela		

- Click on **Return to Nurses' Station**.
- Click on **201** at the bottom of the screen to go to Dorothy Grant's room.
- Click on **Patient Care**.
- Click on **Physical Assessment**.
- Click on **Pelvic** and then on **Reproductive**.

3. Complete the table below with the results of Dorothy Grant's initial cervical examination.

Patient	Time	Dilation	Effacement	Station
Dorothy Grant				

- Click on **Return to Nurses' Station**.
- Click on **205** to go to Gabriela Valenzuela's room.
- Click on **Patient Care**.
- Click on **Physical Assessment**.
- Click on **Pelvic** and then on **Reproductive**.

4. Record the results of Gabriela Valenzuela's initial cervical examination in the table below.

Patient	Time	Dilation	Effacement	Station
Gabriela Valenzuela				

Read the definition of preterm labor on pages 646-657 in your textbook.

5. Preterm labor is defined as the onset of labor after ______________________________

   but before ______________________________.

6. As of Wednesday at 0800, would you consider both these patients to be in preterm labor? Give a rationale for your answer.

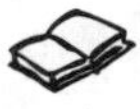

Read the section on Tocolytics on pages 651-653 in your textbook to answer the following questions.

7. Match each medication below with the description of how it works as a tocolytic agent. (*Hint:* Letters may be used more than once.)

Medication

_____ Magnesium sulfate

_____ Nifedipine (Procardia)

_____ Ritodrine (Yutopar)

_____ Terbutaline (Brethine)

_____ Indomethacin (Indocin)

Tocolytic Action

a. Blocks calcium from entering smooth muscle cells, thus relaxing uterine contractions

b. Inhibits uterine muscle activity as a result of stimulation of beta-adrenergic receptors of the sympathetic nervous system

c. Exact mechanism unclear, but promotes relaxation of smooth muscles

d. Suppresses preterm labor by inhibiting the synthesis of prostaglandins

Exercise 2

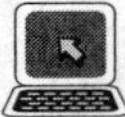

Virtual Hospital Activity

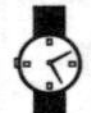

30 minutes

- Sign in to work at Pacific View Regional Hospital on the Obstetrics Floor for Period of Care 1. (*Note*: If you are already in the virtual hospital from a previous exercise, click on **Leave the Floor** and then on **Restart the Program** to get to the sign-in window.)
- From the Patient List, select Stacey Crider.
- Click on **Get Report**.

Stacey Crider was admitted yesterday in preterm labor and given magnesium sulfate. Her other admission diagnoses were bacterial vaginosis and gestational diabetes with poorly controlled blood glucose levels.

1. What is Stacey Crider's current status in regard to preterm labor?

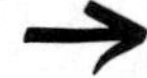

- Click on **Go to Nurses' Station**.
- Click on **Chart** and then on **202**.
- Click on **Physician's Orders**.
- Scroll to the orders for Wednesday at 0715.

2. Which of these orders relate specifically to Stacey Crider's diagnosis of preterm labor?

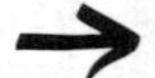

- Scroll to the orders for Wednesday at 0730.

3. What medication changes are ordered?

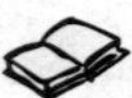 Read about terbutaline on pages 652-653 in your textbook.

4. Why do you think Stacey Crider's physician changed the orders so quickly?

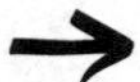

- Click on **Return to Nurses' Station**.
- Click on **202** at the bottom of the screen.
- Inside the patient's room, click on **Take Vital Signs**.

5. What are Stacey Crider's current vital signs?

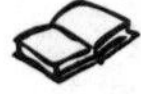

6. Which of these parameters provides you with the most important information before giving Stacey Crider's nifedipine dose? Why? (*Hint*: Read about nifedipine on page 651 in your textbook.)

Like Dorothy Grant and Kelly Brady, Stacey Crider is receiving betamethasone.

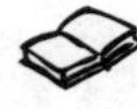 Read the Accelerating Fetal Lung Maturity section in your textbook on pages 653-654. Also consult the Betamethasone, Dexamethasone Drug Guide on page 653. Then answer the following questions.

7. Why are all three of these patients receiving antenatal glucocorticoid therapy?

8. What other benefit does this class of medication seem to provide for preterm infants?

→ • Click on **MAR**.
• Click on tab **202**.

9. What is Stacey Crider's prescribed betamethasone dosage?

10. How does this dosage compare with the recommended dosage in your textbook?

→ • Click on **Return to Nurses' Station**.
• Click on **Medication Room**.
• Click on **Unit Dosage**.
• Click on drawer **202**.
• Click on **Betamethasone**.
• Click on **Put Medication on Tray**.
• Click on **Close Drawer**.
• Click on **View Medication Room**.
• Click on **Preparation**.
• Click on **Prepare** and follow the preparation Wizard's prompts to complete preparation of Stacey Crider's betamethasone dose.
• Click on **Return to Medication Room**.
• Click on **202** to return to Stacey Crider's room.
• Click on **Check Armband**.
• Click on **Check Allergies**.
• Click on **Patient Care**.
• Click on **Medication Administration**.
• Find Betamethasone listed on the left side of your screen. To its right, click on the down arrow next to **Select** and choose **Administer**.
• Follow the Administration Wizard's prompts to administer Stacey Crider's betamethasone injection. Indicate **Yes** to document the injection in the MAR.

- Click on **Leave the Floor**.
- Click on **Look at Your Preceptor's Evaluation**.
- Click on **Medication Scorecard**. How did you do?

Exercise 3

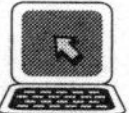

Virtual Hospital Activity

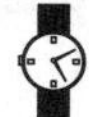

30 minutes

- Sign in to work at Pacific View Regional Hospital on the Obstetrics Floor for Period of Care 4. (*Note*: If you are already in the virtual hospital from a previous exercise, click on **Leave the Floor** and then on **Restart the Program** to get to the sign-in window.)
- From the Nurses' Station, click on **Chart**. (*Remember:* You are not able to visit patients or administer medications during Period of Care 4. You are able to review patient records only.)
- Click on **201** for Dorothy Grant's chart.
- Click on **Nurse's Notes**.
- Scroll to the note for Wednesday 1815.

1. What are the findings from Dorothy Grant's cervical examination at this time?

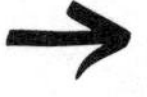

- Scroll to the note for Wednesday 1840. It states that Dorothy Grant is being prepped for delivery.

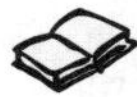

2. If you were the nurse caring for Dorothy Grant during delivery, what special preparations would you make to care for the baby immediately after birth? (*Hint:* Read Teaching What May Occur During a Preterm Birth on page 655 in your textbook.)

- Click on **Return to Nurses' Station**.
- Click again on **Chart**, but this time choose **205** for Gabriela Valenzuela's chart.
- Click on **Physician's Notes** and scroll to the note for Wednesday 0800.

3. What is the anticipated outcome of Gabriela Valenzuela's labor, according to this note?

- Scroll to the notes for Wednesday 1415 and 1455.

4. What preparations have been made during the day for the birth of Gabriela Valenzuela's baby?

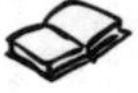 Read the information on cesarean birth found on pages 424-431 in your textbook.

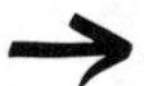

- Click on **Return to Nurses' Station**.
- Click on **Chart** and then on **203**.
- Click on **Physician's Notes**.
- Scroll to the note for Wednesday 1530.

Kelly Brady was admitted yesterday with severe preeclampsia at 26 weeks gestation. Her preeclampsia is now worsening.

5. Why does her physician now recommend immediate delivery?

6. What general risks related to cesarean section does Kelly Brady's physician discuss with her?

7. Because of Kelly Brady's early gestational age (26 weeks), her physician anticipates a classical uterine incision. How will this type of incision affect Kelly Brady's birth options in future pregnancies?

- Click on **Physician's Orders** and scroll to the orders for Wednesday 1540.

8. List the orders to be carried out before Kelly Brady's surgery. State the purpose of each.

Order	Purpose

9. Can you think of other common preoperative procedures? List them below. (*Hint*: Refer to a basic Medical-Surgical textbook for ideas if you need help!)

LESSON 13

Medication Administration

Reading Assignment: Pregnancy-Related Complications (Chapter 25)
Concurrent Disorders During Pregnancy (Chapter 26)
The Woman with Intrapartum Complications (Chapter 27)

Patients: Dorothy Grant, Room 201
Stacey Crider, Room 202
Maggie Gardner, Room 204
Laura Wilson, Room 206

Goal: Correctly administer selected medications to obstetric patients.

Objective:

1. Correctly administer selected medications to obstetric patients, observing the six rights.

Exercise 1

Virtual Hospital Activity

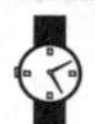

30 minutes

Dorothy Grant was admitted at 30 weeks gestation for observation following blunt abdominal trauma (she was kicked in the abdomen). She is bleeding vaginally and may have sustained a placental abruption. Your assignment is to give Rho(D) immune globulin to her.

- Sign in to work at Pacific View Regional Hospital on the Obstetrics Floor for Period of Care 2. (*Note*: If you are already in the virtual hospital from a previous exercise, click on **Leave the Floor** and then on **Restart the Program** to get to the sign-in window.)
- From the Patient List, select Dorothy Grant.

Read about Rho(D) immune globulin on page 603 in your textbook.

1. Rho(D) immune globulin is given to prevent ______________________________

   in Rh-______________ women who have been exposed to Rh-______________ blood.

   Rho(D) immune globulin suppresses the ______________________________

   ____.

2. All of the following are reasons that Rho(D) immune globulin might be administered. Select the reason it has been ordered for Dorothy Grant.

_____ Within 72 hours of giving birth to an Rh-positive infant

_____ Prophylactically at 28 weeks gestation

_____ Following an incident or exposure risk that occurs after 28 weeks gestation

_____ During first trimester pregnancy following miscarriage or elective abortion or ectopic pregnancy

3. List the information about Dorothy Grant that must be determined before giving her Rho(D) immune globulin.

→ • Click on **Go to Nurses' Station**.
• Click on **Chart** and then on **201**.
• Click on **Physician's Orders** and scroll to the orders for Wednesday 0730.

4. Write the physician's order for Rho(D) immune globulin.

5. According to your textbook, is this the correct dosage and route? (*Hint:* Read the section on Postpartum Management on page 603-604 in your textbook.)

→ • Click on **Laboratory Reports**.
• Locate the results for 0245 Wednesday.
• Scroll down to find the type and screen results.

6. Dorothy Grant's blood type is ______________________.

7. What additional information do you need? Why? Is that information available?

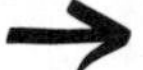

- Click on **Return to Nurses' Station**.
- Click on **Medication Room**.
- Click on **Refrigerator**; then click on the refrigerator door to open it.
- Click on **Put Medication on Tray**.
- Click on **Close Door**.
- Click on **View Medication Room**.
- Click on **Preparation**.
- Click on **Prepare** and follow the prompts to complete preparation of this medication.
- Click on **Return to Medication Room**.
- Click on **201** to go to Dorothy Grant's room.
- Click on **Check Armband**.
- Click on **Patient Care**.
- Click on **Medication Administration**.

You are almost ready to give Dorothy Grant's injection. However, before you do . . .

8. Rho(D) immune globulin is often considered a blood product.
   a. True
   b. False

9. Suppose Dorothy Grant absolutely refuses to accept blood or blood products because of her religious beliefs. How would you handle the situation?

Now you're ready to administer the medication!

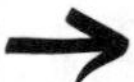

- Click on the down arrow next to **Select**; choose **Administer**.
- Follow the prompts to administer Dorothy Grant's injection. Indicate **Yes** to document the injection in the MAR.
- Click on **Leave the Floor**.
- Click on **Look at Your Preceptor's Evaluation**.
- Click on **Medication Scorecard**. How did you do?

Exercise 2

Virtual Hospital Activity

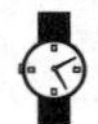

20 minutes

- Sign in to work at Pacific View Regional Hospital on the Obstetrics Floor for Period of Care 1. (*Note*: If you are already in the virtual hospital from a previous exercise, click on **Leave the Floor** and then on **Restart the Program** to get to the sign-in window.)
- From the Patient List, select Maggie Gardner.
- Click on **Go to Nurses' Station**.
- Click on the **Chart** and then on **204**.
- Click on the **Nursing Admission**.

1. Maggie Gardner verbalizes anxiety repeatedly throughout the Nursing Admission. What is her primary concern? Why? Provide documentation.

2. Maggie Gardner states that before this pregnancy, she had a highly adaptive coping mechanism. How does she consider her ability to cope at this point? Why? (*Hint*: See the Coping and Stress Tolerance section in the Nursing Admission.)

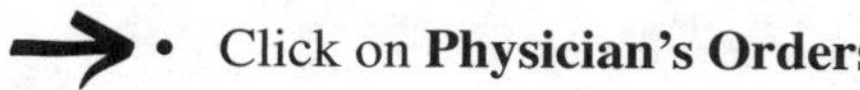

- Click on **Physician's Orders**.

3. What medication has the physician ordered to help Maggie Gardner with her anxiety?

- Click on **Return to Nurses' Station**.
- Click on the **Drug** icon in the lower-left corner of your screen.
- Use the search box or the scroll bar to find the medication you identified in question 3.
- Review all of the information provided regarding this drug.

4. What is the drug's mechanism of action?

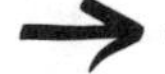

- Click on **Return to Nurses' Station**.
- Click on **204** to go to Maggie Gardner's room.
- Click on **Patient Care** and then on **Nurse-Client Interactions**.
- Select and view the video titled **0745: Evaluation—Efficacy of Drugs**. (*Note*: Check the virtual clock to see whether enough time has elapsed. You can use the fast-forward feature to advance the time by 2-minute intervals if the video is not yet available. Then click again on **Patient Care** and **Nurse-Client Interactions** to refresh the screen.)

5. According to the nurse, how long will it take for Maggie Gardner to see therapeutic effects of the medication that has been ordered? How does this correlate with what you learned in the Teaching Section of the Drug Guide?

Exercise 3

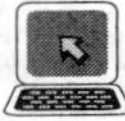

Virtual Hospital Activity

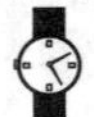

15 minutes

In this exercise, you will administer betamethasone to Stacey Crider, who was admitted to the hospital at 27 weeks gestation in preterm labor.

- Sign in to work at Pacific View Regional Hospital on the Obstetrics Floor for Period of Care 1. (*Note*: If you are already in the virtual hospital from a previous exercise, click on **Leave the Floor** and then on **Restart the Program** to get to the sign-in window.)
- From the Patient List, select Stacey Crider.

1. Before preparing Stacey Crider's betamethasone, what do you need to do first?

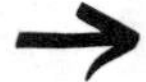

- Click on **Go to Nurses' Station**.
- Click on **Chart** and then on **202**.
- Click on **Physician's Orders**.
- Scroll until you find the order for betamethasone.

2. After verifying the physician's order, what is your next step?

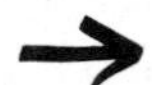

- Click on **Return to Nurses' Station**.
- Click on **Medication Room**.
- Click on **Unit Dosage**.
- Click on drawer **202**.
- Click on **Betamethasone**.
- Click on **Put Medication on Tray**.
- Click on **Close Drawer**.
- Click on **View Medication Room**.
- Click on **Preparation**.
- Click on **Prepare** and follow the prompts to complete preparation of Stacey Crider's betamethasone dose.
- Click on **Return to Medication Room**.

3. Now that the medication is prepared, what is your next step?

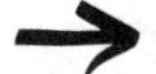

- Click on **202** to go to the patient's room.
- Click on **Check Armband**.
- Click on **Check Allergies**.
- Click on **Patient Care**.
- Click on **Medication Administration**.
- Click on the down arrow next to **Select** and choose **Administer**.
- Follow the prompts to administer Stacey Crider's betamethasone injection.

4. What is the final step in the process?

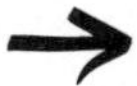

- If you haven't already done so, indicate **Yes** to document the injection in the MAR.
- Click on **Leave the Floor**.
- Click on **Look at Your Preceptor's Evaluation**.
- Click on **Medication Scorecard**. How did you do?

Exercise 4

Virtual Hospital Activity

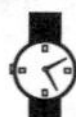

30 minutes

- Sign in to work at Pacific View Regional Hospital on the Obstetrics Floor for Period of Care 1. (*Note*: If you are already in the virtual hospital from a previous exercise, click on **Leave the Floor** and then on **Restart the Program** to get to the sign-in window.)
- From the Patient List, select Laura Wilson.
- Click on **Go to Nurses' Station**.
- Click on **MAR**.
- Click on the tab for **206**.

1. Laura Wilson's medications for Wednesday include several different types of drugs. In the list below, select the one that is used to treat her HIV-positive status.

_____ Zidovudine 200 mg PO every 8 hours

_____ Prenatal multivitamin 1 tablet PO daily

_____ Lactated Ringer's solution 1000 mL IV continuous

- Click on **Return to Nurses' Station**.
- Click on the **Drug** icon in the lower-left corner of the screen.
- Using the search box or the scroll bar, find the drug you identified in question 1.

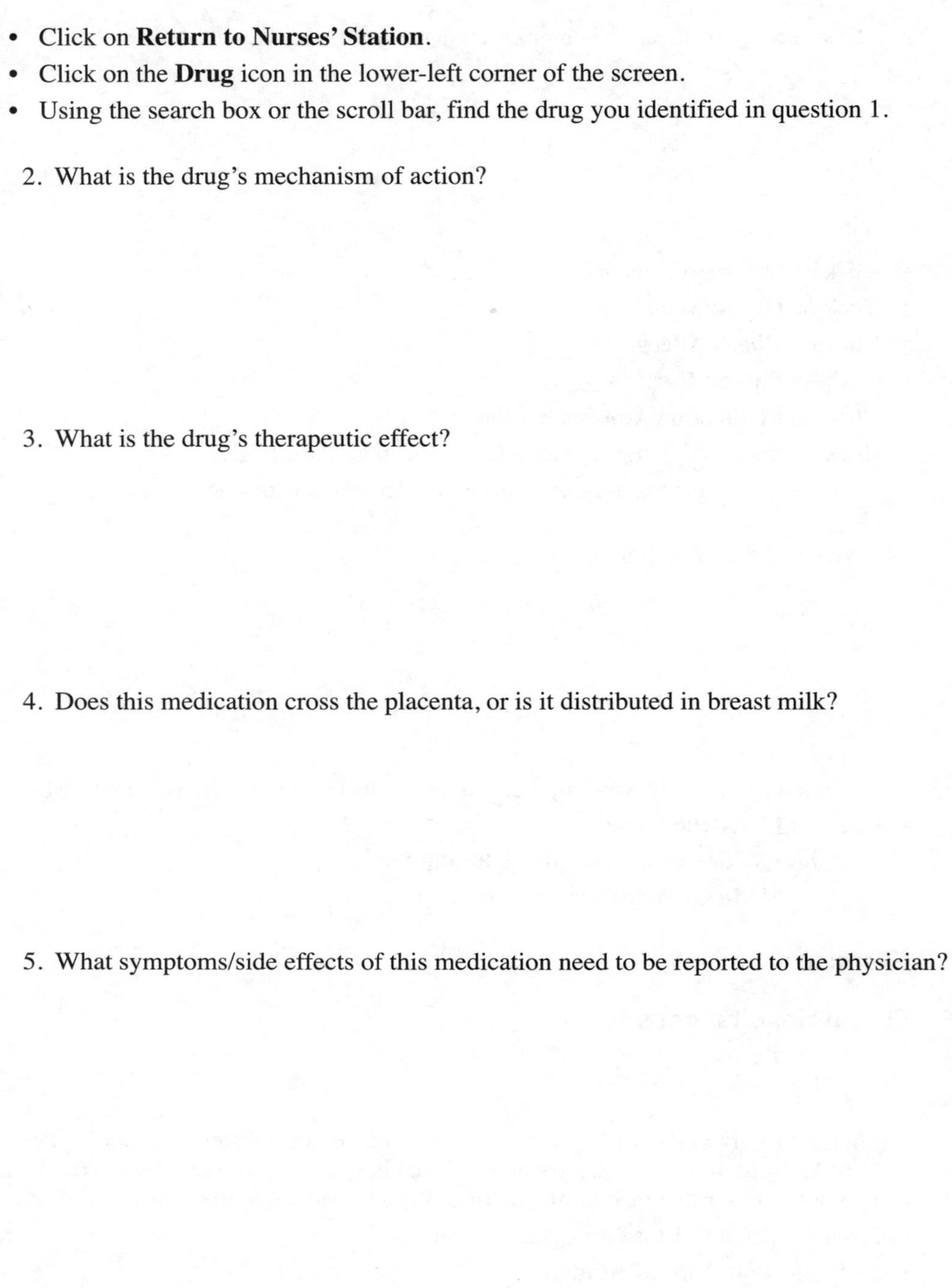

2. What is the drug's mechanism of action?

3. What is the drug's therapeutic effect?

4. Does this medication cross the placenta, or is it distributed in breast milk?

5. What symptoms/side effects of this medication need to be reported to the physician?

6. How should this medication be taken?

7. Your final assignment dealing with obstetric patients is to give Laura Wilson the medication that is due at 0800. During these lessons, we have provided you with the detailed instructions on how to give medications. Now it is time for you to try this on your own. Don't forget the six rights of medication administration. Document below how you did.

If you'd like to get more practice, there are other medications that can be given at the beginning of the first three periods of care. Below is a list of the patients, the medications, the routes of administration, and the administration times you can use. As you practice, be sure to select the correct patient when you sign in. That way, you can get a Medication Scorecard for evaluation after you prepare and administer a medication. (*Remember:* If you need help at any time, refer to pages 22, 26-30, and 37-41 in the **Getting Started** section of this workbook.)

PERIOD OF CARE 1

Room 201, Dorothy Grant

0730/0800: Betamethasone 12 mg IM

Prenatal multivitamin PO

Room 202, Stacey Crider

0800: Prenatal multivitamin PO

Metronidazole 500 mg PO

Betamethasone 12 mg IM

Insulin lispro subQ

Nifedipine 20 mg PO

Room 203, Kelly Brady

0730/0800: Prenatal multivitamin PO

Ferrous sulfate PO

Labetalol hydrochloride 400 mg PO

Nifedipine 10 mg PO

Room 204, Maggie Gardner

0800: Prenatal multivitamin PO

Buspirone hydrochloride 5 mg PO

Room 205, Gabriela Valenzuela

0800: Ampicillin 2 g IV

Betamethasone 12 mg IM

Prenatal multivitamin PO

Room 206, Laura Wilson

0800: Zidovudine 200 mg PO

Prenatal multivitamin PO

PERIOD OF CARE 2

Room 201, Dorothy Grant

1200: Rho(D) immune globulin IM

Room 202, Stacey Crider

1200: Insulin lispro subQ

Room 203, Kelly Brady

1130: Betamethasone 12 mg IM

Room 204, Maggie Gardner

1115: Prednisone 40 mg PO

Aspirin 81 mg PO

PERIOD OF CARE 3

Room 204, Maggie Gardner

1500: Buspirone 5 mg PO

LESSON 14

Caring for an Infant with Bronchiolitis

Reading Assignment: Health Promotion for the Infant (Chapter 6)
Principles and Procedures for Nursing Care of Children (Chapter 37, pages 938-941)
The Child with a Respiratory Alteration (Chapter 45, pages 1146-1148, 1165-1167)

Patient: Carrie Richards, Room 303

Goal: Demonstrate an understanding of nursing care for an infant with bronchiolitis.

Objectives:

1. Discuss etiology and pathophysiology of bronchiolitis.
2. Relate the effect of an infant's level of growth and development on bronchiolitis.
3. Complete a respiratory assessment on an infant and discuss nursing care issues.
4. Use the nursing process to develop a nursing care plan for an infant with bronchiolitis.

Exercise 1

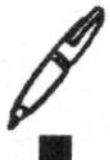

Writing Activity

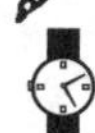

15 minutes

1. Explain the pathophysiology of bronchiolitis.

- edema & accumulation of mucus & cellular debris causes obstruction of the bronchioles.
- mild URT infection usually precedes the development of bronchiolitis
- child will have: serous nasal drainage, sneezing, low-grade fever, & anorexia present for several days. This is then followed by onset of acute respiratory distress with the signs & symptos of: tachypnea (rr 60-80), tachycardia (hr greater 140), wheezing, crackles, or rhonchi cyanosis, intercostal & subcostal retractions ē or ēout nasal flaring temperature varies from hypothermic to as high as 41°c

2. Explain the relationship of respiratory syncytial virus (RSV) to bronchiolitis.

A upper respiratory tract infection usually precedes the development of bronchiolitis. RSV is the causative agent in more than half of cases.

3. Discuss the effect of Carrie Richards' growth and development on her diagnosis of bronchiolitis.

-around 3 and a half months babies start to roll over. having ↓ energy and ↑ WOB could delay this mile stone slightly. Also bronchiolitis could put Carrie at risk for developing asthma

4. Think about how you would explain a diagnosis of bronchiolitis to Carrie Richards' mother. What information would you share? How would you present it?

The bronchioles are blocked by muccus and inflamatin which is why Carrie is on oxygen, sats monitor, and head needs to be elevated! 30-40° That Carrie is most acutely ill during the first 48-72 hrs. and should improve after a few days. However her symptoms may last for 10-14 days.

Exercise 2

Virtual Hospital Activity

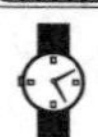

30 minutes

- Sign in to work at Pacific View Regional Hospital on the Pediatrics Floor for Period of Care 1. (*Note:* If you are already in the virtual hospital from a previous exercise, click on **Leave the Floor** and then on **Restart the Program** to get to the sign-in window.)
- From the Patient List, select Carrie Richards.
- Click on **Go to Nurses' Station**.
- Click on **Chart** and then on **303**.
- Click on **Emergency Department** and review this record.
- Click on and review the **Physician's Orders**, **History and Physical**, and **Nursing Admission**.

1. As you read these records, list the data that are consistent with bronchiolitis.

rr=56 p=155 T: 99°F
substernal retraction flaring
cap refil >4sec
wheeze, crackles, labored resps.
Skin turgor ↓
urin output ↓
pulse ox 88-89 on RA

2. Refer to the Physician's Orders. What is the rationale for the orders for IV fluid, medications, oxygen, pulse oximetry, and lab work?

IV: to help c̄ dehydration & risk for aspiration

meds: - Albuterol
- Racemic epinephrine
help with breathing

O2: to keep Stas > 92%

lab: - CBC: check for infection
- urinalysis: to check for glucos & infection
- arterial blood gas: to check oxygenation levels
- serum chem, electrolyts: check nutritional deficit
- chest xray: show hyperinflation of the lungs & ↑ anteroposterior chest diamater on lateral view

3. Carrie Richards had nasal washing done while she was in the Emergency Department. If you were performing the nasal washing procedure, would you anticipate restraining her? If so, how? Would you have Carrie Richards' mother help? What factors would you consider to help you decide what to do? (*Hint:* Check Carrie's physical status and behavior while in the Emergency Department.)

Yes I would anticipate restraining her because nasal washing is a uncomfortable procedure. I would mummy wrap Carrie. I wouldn't have Carrie's mother help, so Carrie doesn't associate her with the procedure

4. Explain the type of isolation being used. (*Hint:* To find this, check the Physician's Orders.) What other infection control precautions need to be implemented?

The isolation being used is contact isolation. This type of isolation requires anyone to wear gloves, gown, and follow strict hand hygine. Carrie should be put in a private room or a room with a nother child that has RSV.

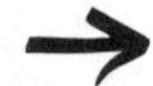

- Click on **Return to Nurses' Station** and then on **303** at the bottom of the screen.
- Click on **Patient Care** and then on **Nurse-Client Interactions**.
- Select and view the video titled **0730: Patient Assessment**. (*Note*: Check the virtual clock to see whether enough time has elapsed. You can use the fast-forward feature to advance the time by 2-minute intervals if the video is not yet available. Then click again on **Patient Care** and **Nurse-Client Interactions** to refresh the screen.)

5. During the video, did you notice any infection control precautions that where incorrect? If so, explain.

↳ mask
↳ gown
↳ gloves

The nurse & mom were wearing masks. Contact precaution doesn't require a mask because the illness isn't transmitted in the air.

Exercise 3

Virtual Hospital Activity

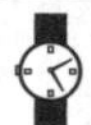

45 minutes

- Sign in to work at Pacific View Regional Hospital on the Pediatrics Floor for Period of Care 1. (*Note:* If you are already in the virtual hospital from a previous exercise, click on **Leave the Floor** and then on **Restart the Program** to get to the sign-in window.)
- From the Patient List, select Carrie Richards.
- Click on **Go to Nurses' Station**.
- Click on **303** to go to Carrie's room.
- Inside the room, click on **Check Armband** and then on **Take Vital Signs**. Note Carrie's vital signs for documentation. BP 91/53 sats 95% T: 99.2 HR 124 rr 44 CL on 2L
- Next, click on **Patient Care** and do a head-to-toe assessment by clicking on the various body system categories and subcategories. Take notes as needed.

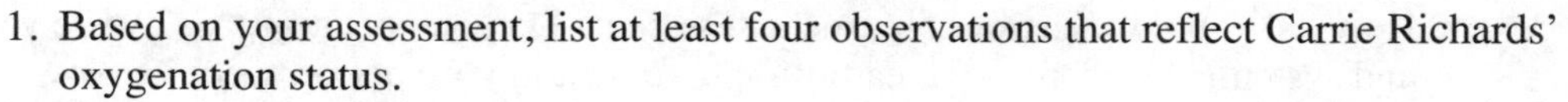

1. Based on your assessment, list at least four observations that reflect Carrie Richards' oxygenation status.

- skin color
- O_2 sats
- O_2 need
- breath sounds

2. Carrie Richards is of African-American descent. What is the best way to assess her color?

check her oral mucosa and nail beds.

- Click on **EPR** and then on **Login**.
- Specify **303** from the Patient drop-down menu and **Vital Signs** from the Category drop-down menu. Use the blue arrows as needed to scroll and document the data you collected in the appropriate time column.
- Continue to chart your observations in the **Respiratory** and **Cardiovascular** categories.

3. If you missed anything, go back to Carrie Richards' room and reassess her. Because the EPR format is generic, you may not have data for all areas listed. You do, however, need to make sure you are recognizing significant assessment data. Review data trends since admission. What is your assessment of Carrie Richards' status? Why is continued monitoring necessary?

Carrie Richards' status is improving. Continued monitoring is necessary to identifily any negative changes quickly and interven as appropriate.

4. How did you do with your focused assessment? Do you note any gaps? Were you efficient and systemic? Is there any area for improvement in your performance?

Answer the following questions based on your assessment findings.

5. Is Carrie Richards' condition improving or deteriorating?

Carrie Richards' condition is improving.

6. List some changes that might occur if Carrie Richards' condition were deteriorating.

- ↑ Oxygen needs
- persistant fever
- ↑ heart rate and WOB

7. Carrie Richards is receiving oxygen via a nasal cannula.

8. Sometimes oxygen is delivered in a mist tent. What are the nursing responsibilities for care of an infant in a mist tent? Are there any advantages to using a mist tent rather than a nasal cannula? Or vice versa?

-Keep the child as dry as possible
-use cotton clothing
-Δ clothing and beding as needed
-ensure all sides of the tent are compllatly tucked in to prevent escape of oxygen
The mist tent is used when only moisture & minimal oxygen is needed.
Nasal cannulas are used when more concentrated oxygen is required.

9. Carrie Richards' O_2 status is being monitored by a pulse oximeter.

The device should be attached to Carrie Richards' toe.

Persistent levels below 92% should be reported.

10. Which of the following should be included when documenting observations associated with Carrie Richards' O_2 saturation levels? Select all that apply.

✓ Response to specific activity

✓ A comparative assessment of oxygenation status

✓ Whether Carrie Richards was receiving O_2 or on room air

11. Oxygenation assessment is ongoing. In older children and adults, the nurse can easily assess respiratory status in response to play or other activity. How can this ongoing assessment be carried out in an infant?

Ask the parents what the infant normaly does and compair this to what the infant is doing

Exercise 4

Writing Activity

20 minutes

1. You have completed an oxygenation assessment. Write the priority nursing diagnosis with the expected outcome for Carrie Richards based on the textbook information. How does this compare with Carrie Richards' care plan in her Kardex?

Impaired gas exchoge related to airway edema and increased mucus. Expected outcome: The infant will have adequate gas exchange, as evidenced by oxygen saturation above 95% on room air.
* Carrie's care plan main focuse is on nutrition and mother baby bonding

2. Based on your textbook readings, list three other nursing diagnoses with their expected outcomes.

- Deficient Fluid volume related to decreased intake and insensible loss. Expected outcome: the infant will maintain adequate hydration as evidenced by moist mucous membranes, a flat Fontanel, urine output normal for age, & stable weight.
- Ineffective airway clearance related to ↑ secretions. Expected outcome: the infant will exhibit clear breath sounds & normal resp. rate, depth, & rhythm
- Ineffective thermoregulation related to illness. Expected outcome: The infant will demonstrate a body temp with in normal limits.

3. List at least thee areas of teaching that could be completed with Carrie Richards' mother related to the diagnosis of bronchiolitis.

- how to use a bulb syringe to suction Carrie's nares.
- how to perform chest physio
- Signs and symptoms of a RSV recurance

LESSON 15

Nursing Care Issues Associated with Bronchiolitis

Reading Assignment: Health Promotion for the Infant (Chapter 6)
Medication Administration and Safety for Infants and Children (Chapter 38, pages 948-955 and 960-966)
The Child with a Fluid and Electrolyte Alteration (Chapter 40, pages 989-999)
The Child with a Developmental Disability (Chapter 54, pages 1493-1494)

Patient: Carrie Richards, Room 303

Goal: Demonstrate an understanding of other problems and care issues associated with bronchiolitis.

Objectives:

1. Discuss the reasons why infants are at risk for hydration problems.
2. Explain the risk for dehydration in infants with respiratory problems.
3. Discuss nursing care for managing hydration concerns, including intravenous (IV) therapy.
4. Discuss nutritional needs of the infant.
5. Differentiate between organic and nonorganic failure to thrive.
6. Explore assessment required when failure to thrive is suspected.
7. Identify and discuss areas for independent teaching in the care of infants.
8. Discuss discharge teaching responsibilities for the patient with bronchiolitis, dehydration, and failure to thrive.

Exercise 1

Virtual Hospital Activity

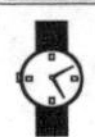

45 minutes

1. List the characteristics of infants that put them at greater risk for hydration problems. Place an asterisk next to those that particularly relate to dehydration as a potential problem with respiratory illness.

2. Which of the following hydration assessments used with Carrie Richards would not be available with an older child?
   a. Weight
   b. Skin turgor
   c. Vital signs
   d. Anterior fontanel
   e. Presence of tears
   f. Eyes
   g. Mucous membranes
   h. Capillary refill
   i. Intake and output

- Sign in to work at Pacific View Regional Hospital on the Pediatrics Floor for Period of Care 1. (*Note:* If you are already in the virtual hospital from a previous exercise, click on **Leave the Floor** and then on **Restart the Program** to get to the sign-in window.)
- From the Patient List, select Carrie Richards.
- Click on **Get Report** and then on **Go to Nurses' Station**.
- Click on **303** at the bottom of your screen.
- Click on **Patient Care** and complete a focused assessment of Carrie Richards. (*Remember:* A focused assessment is one that addresses the priority health concern as well as those concerns for which the patient is at risk.)
- Once your assessment is complete, click on **EPR** and then on **Login**.
- Specify Carrie Richards' room number (**303**) and choose categories as needed to record the data from your focused assessment. (*Hint:* If you need help entering data in the EPR, refer to pages 15-16 in the **Getting Started** section of this workbook.)
- When you have finished documenting your assessments, click on **Exit EPR**.
- Now, to see how you did, click on **Leave the Floor**.
- From the Floor Menu, select **Look at Your Preceptor's Evaluations**.
- Now click on **Examination Report** and review the feedback.

3. Summarize your performance with this assessment. Did you include an assessment of the respiratory status along with hydration parameters?

4. What is the most reliable information you can use to assess an infant's hydration over time? Why?

5. Discuss the nursing responsibilities associated with IV fluid administration in infants. (*Hint:* Remember that IV fluid is treated as a medication administration.)

6. What should the nurse be looking for when assessing an IV site?

7. You find that infusion pumps are in very short supply. You know that Carrie Richards, because of her age, needs a pump and will get the next available one. In the meantime, you must anticipate using IV tubing that has a burette. What is the rationale for use of this type of tubing?

→ • Click on **Chart** and then on **303**.
• Click on **Nursing Admissions**.

8. Calculate Carrie Richards' daily fluid maintenance needs. (*Hint:* You will need to find her weight in the Nursing Admission form to make this calculation.)

9. What would you tell Carrie Richards' mother about adequate hydration? How she will know whether her baby is getting enough fluids?

→ • Now click on **Physician's Orders**. Find the most recent order for IV fluids for Carrie.

10. Carrie Richards is receiving an IV infusion with potassium added. Explain what she is receiving. Discuss the nurse's responsibilities related to potassium administration to an infant.

11. Consider what aspects of care (with regard to managing the IV) you may delegate to Carrie Richards' mother. What could you ask her to do while still maintaining safe care and fulfilling your legal responsibility?

Exercise 2

Virtual Hospital Activity

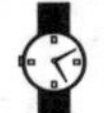

30 minutes

- Sign in to work at Pacific View Regional Hospital on the Pediatrics Floor for Period of Care 3. (*Note:* If you are already in the virtual hospital from a previous exercise, click on **Leave the Floor** and then on **Restart the Program** to get to the sign-in window.)
- From the Patient List, select Carrie Richards.
- Click on **Go to Nurses' Station**.
- Click on **303** to go to Carrie's room.
- Click on **Take Vital Signs**.
- Click on **Clinical Alerts** and review the report.

1. Can Carrie Richards have acetaminophen? If so, for what reason will you be giving it?

2. What should you assess or check before you prepare the medication? (*Hint:* Consider the specific need for this medication, as well as the nursing responsibilities before administering any medication.)

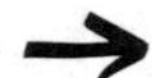

- Click on **MAR** and find the order for this medication.

3. Is the ordered dose of this medication appropriate for Carrie Richards? If not, why not? Include your calculations to support your answer.

4. What are the appropriate methods for administering oral medications to an infant?

- Click on **Return to Room 303**.
- Click on **Medication Room**.
- Click on **Unit Dosage**.
- Click on drawer **303**.
- Click on **Acetaminophen**.
- Click on **Put Medication on Tray**.
- Click on **Close Drawer**.
- Click on **View Medication Room**.
- Click on **Preparation**.
- Click on **Prepare** and follow the Preparation Wizard's prompts to complete preparation of Carrie's acetaminophen dose.
- Click on **Return to Medication Room**.
- Click on **303** to return to Carrie's room.
- Click on **Check Armband**.
- Click on **Check Allergies**.
- Click on **Patient Care**.
- Click on **Medication Administration**.
- Find **Acetaminophen** listed on the left side of your screen. To its right, click on the down arrow next to **Select** and choose **Administer**.
- Follow the Administration Wizard's prompts to administer the medication. Indicate **Yes** to document the injection in the MAR.
- Click on **Leave the Floor**.
- Click on **Look at Your Preceptor's Evaluation**.
- Click on **Medication Scorecard**. How did you do?

5. Now that you have administered the acetaminophen, what side effects would be evidence of a negative reaction to the medication? (*Hint:* See the Drug Guide for help.)

You have just been walked through the medication preparation and administration procedure. Now try it on your own. To do so, you have two options:

- Click on **MAR** and see whether Carrie Richards has any other medications due at this time. If she does, you can stay in this period of care and proceed with the preparation and administration.
- If you prefer to practice preparing and giving Carrie Richards the same acetaminophen dose you just completed, click on **Leave the Floor** and then on **Restart the Program**. Sign in again to work with Carrie for Period of Care 3 and proceed from there.

Regardless of which option you choose, remember to follow the six rights! After you have finished administering the medication, be sure to see how you did by checking your Medication Scorecard.

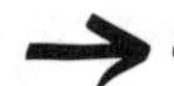

- Click on **Leave the Floor** and then on **Look at Your Preceptor's Evaluations**.
- Click on **Medication Scorecard** and review your evaluation.

6. Carrie Richards' mother needs to know how to give her infant medication at home. How will you determine whether she is skillful and comfortable enough giving her baby medication?

7. How would you respond to the following concern: "The nurse is supposed to give the medication, so how can the nurse allow a parent to administer medication?" (*Hint:* To answer this, you need to think through the nurse's legal responsibilities.)

Exercise 3

Writing Activity

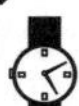

10 minutes

1. What topics would you include in Carrie Richards' discharge instructions after hospitalization with bronchiolitis?

2. What will you do to ensure teaching is understood?

3. Providing anticipatory guidance is very important. Carrie Richards is 3½ months old. Identify some changes her mother should anticipate in the next few weeks.

Exercise 4

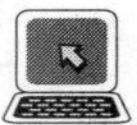

Virtual Hospital Activity

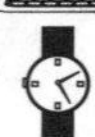

10 minutes

- Sign in to work at Pacific View Regional Hospital on the Pediatrics Floor for Period of Care 1. (*Note:* If you are already in the virtual hospital from a previous exercise, click on **Leave the Floor** and then on **Restart the Program** to get to the sign-in window.)
- From the Patient List, select Carrie Richards.
- Click on **Go to Nurses' Station**.
- Click on **Chart** and then on **303**.
- Click on and review the **History and Physical**.

1. Why is adequate nutrition so important in infancy?

2. At 3½ months of age, Carrie Richards should be receiving _________ ounces of formula _________ times per day.

3. Match each of the following terms with its correct description.

Term	Description
_____ Organic failure to thrive	a. A condition characterized by failure to gain weight secondary to physical factors, such as a gastrointestinal disorder or a metabolic disorder
_____ Nonorganic failure to thrive	b. A condition in which environmental factors influence the intake of calories

4. The following is a list of assessment data. Decide which of these data specifically apply to Carrie Richards based on your review of the chart. Select all that apply.

_____ Weight less than 5th percentile

_____ Sudden deceleration in growth

_____ Delay in reaching milestones

_____ Decreased muscle mass

_____ Muscle hypotonia

_____ Abdominal distention

_____ General weakness

_____ Cachexia

_____ Avoidance of eye contact or touch

_____ Intense watchfulness

_____ Sleep disturbance

_____ Lack of age-appropriate stranger anxiety

_____ Lack of preference for parents

_____ Repetitive self-stimulating behavior

Exercise 5

Virtual Hospital Activity

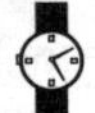

10 minutes

- Sign in to work at Pacific View Regional Hospital on the Pediatrics Floor for Period of Care 2. (*Note:* If you are already in the virtual hospital from a previous exercise, click on **Leave the Floor** and then on **Restart the Program** to get to the sign-in window.)
- From the Patient List, select Carrie Richards.
- Click on **Go to Nurses' Station**.
- Click on **Chart** and then on **303**.
- Click on **Nursing Admission**.

1. Review Carrie Richards' chart for growth information. Plot her length and weight on the growth chart found in your textbook. In what percentile does Carrie fall?

2. With normal growth, there is a doubling of birth weight at about _____ months and a

   ____________________ at 12 months.

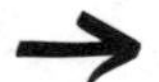

- Now click on **Consultations**.
- Review the Dietary/Nutrition Consult.

3. Find Carrie Richards' birth weight. Based on this information, what concerns do you have about her rate of growth?

4. Based on your review of the Dietary/Nutrition Consult, what do you think is the problem in regard to Carrie Richards' feedings? What additional dietary recommendations are planned for her?

5. As you talk with Carrie Richards' mother, you learn that income is a problem. When discussing feeding, what interdisciplinary collaboration should take place? What are the potential outcomes when taking this approach?

T 102.6 P 126 R 20 BP 107/62 wt 26 lb 11.8 kg

drowsy vomiting, severe headache started 2300 fever 104

pupils Ⓛ Ⓡ 4 4 glasgow 15 O2 sats 98%

urin ↓

+ brudzinski & Kernig

neg bleedn rash photophobia

glucos 191 K 3.0 Na 132

@ 2.5 yrs hit head

head hurt 3/5

sleepy easy aroused

LESSON 16

Caring for a Young Child with Meningitis

Reading Assignment: Health Promotion During Early Childhood (Chapter 7)
Pain Management for Children (Chapter 39, pages 981-982)
The Child with a Neurologic Alteration
(Chapter 52, pages 1411-1418 and 1438-1441)

Patient: Stephanie Brown, Room 304

Goal: Demonstrate an understanding of nursing care for a child with meningitis.

Objectives:

1. Describe the pathophysiology of meningitis.
2. Discuss risk factors for meningitis.
3. List assessment data indicative of meningitis.
4. Explain the rationale for the treatment of meningitis.
5. Develop a care plan for a child with meningitis.
6. Discuss strategies for supporting a parent and child through diagnosis and treatment.

Exercise 1

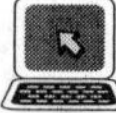

Virtual Hospital Activity

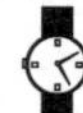

30 minutes

- Sign in to work at Pacific View Regional Hospital on the Pediatrics Floor for Period of Care 1. (*Note:* If you are already in the virtual hospital from a previous exercise, click on **Leave the Floor** and then on **Restart the Program** to get to the sign-in window.)
- From the Patient List, select Stephanie Brown.
- Click on **Get Report**.
- Click on **Go to Nurses' Station**.
- Click on **Chart** and then on **304**.
- Review the following sections of the chart: **Physician's Notes**, **Emergency Department**, **History and Physical**, and **Nursing Admission**.

1. What elements of Stephanie Brown's situation increase her risk for developing meningitis?

2. What assessment data on admissions did Stephanie Brown exhibit that would indicate a diagnosis of meningitis?

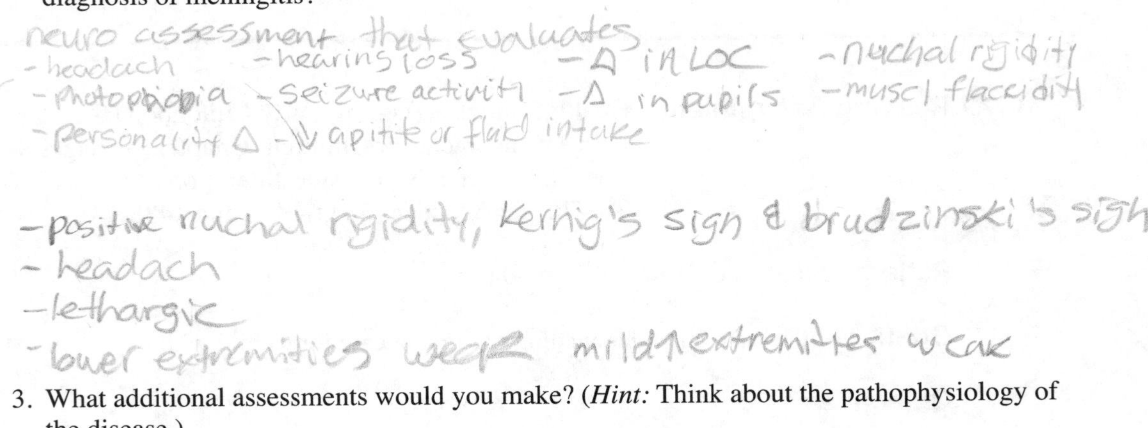

3. What additional assessments would you make? (*Hint:* Think about the pathophysiology of the disease.)

4. If Stephanie Brown were 3 months old and had this diagnosis, what other assessments could you perform?

5. In addition to nuchal rigidity, positive responses to two other signs were elicited from Stephanie Brown that are indicative of meningitis. They are brudzinski's and kernig's signs.

6. Explain how each of the signs listed below is tested. Then briefly describe the response each sign would elicit in a child with meningitis.

Sign	To Test for Sign	Response in Meningitis
Nuchal rigidity (stiff neck)	flexion of the head	any attempt of flexion is difficult. forceful flexion causes severe pain
Kernig's sign	The child can easily extend the leg when in supine position when thigh is flexed towards and pain prevents comple extension of the leg	
Brudzinski's sign	In supine position the child bends head toward chest	This action usualy produces involuntary hip & knee flextion

- Still in Stephanie Brown's chart, click on **Physician's Orders** and review.
- Then click on **Diagnostic Reports** and review.

7. The testing of CSF obtained from a lumbar puncture yields information as to whether meningitis is present or not. Characteristics that are indicative of meningitis include cloudy cerebral spinal fluid (if bacterial), increased protein, low glucose, and increased pressure.

8. Match each of the following physician's orders with its rationale.

	Physician's Order	Rationale
g	Pulse oximetry q4h	a. To establish baseline (aminoglycosides can cause ototoxicity)
d	Neuro checks q4h	b. To utilize gravity in reducing intracranial pressure
f	Blood culture for fever above 101 degrees	c. To maintain therapeutic blood level
a	Audiogram	d. To monitor neurologic status
b	Keep HOB elevated 45 degrees	e. To prevent transmission of disease via droplets
e	Respiratory isolation	f. To assess for other causative agents
c	Vancomycin levels	g. To perform ongoing monitoring of O_2 status

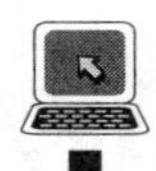

Exercise 2

Virtual Hospital Activity

45 minutes

- Sign in to work at Pacific View Regional Hospital on the Pediatrics Floor for Period of Care 1. (*Note:* If you are already in the virtual hospital from a previous exercise, click on **Leave the Floor** and then on **Restart the Program** to get to the sign-in window.)
- From the Patient List, select Stephanie Brown.
- Click on **Go to Nurses' Station** and then on **304**.
- Click on **Patient Care** and then on **Nurse-Client Interactions**.
- Select and view the video titled **0730: Assessment—Neuro Status**. (*Note*: Check the virtual clock to see whether enough time has elapsed. You can use the fast-forward feature to advance the time by 2-minute intervals if the video is not yet available. Then click again on **Patient Care** and **Nurse-Client Interactions** to refresh the screen.)

1. The isolation guidelines are implemented immediately and kept in place until 24 hours after antibiotics have been started. Antibiotics are always administered before the cultures come back. Why?

It could take up to 3 days to yield results and a delay in treatment could be fatal

-wearing mask & gown no gloves

2. What kind of isolation was the nurse in the video using? Was this correct and consistent with the physician's orders?

The nurse is using droplet precautions this is correct & consistent with physician's orders

3. Suppose that you see Stephanie Brown's mother not wearing a mask. When you ask her about this, she says she doesn't need to do anything special because she never leaves Stephanie's room. How would you respond?

Educate the mother that because meningitis is transmitted by droplet and we don't know the kind of infection She is at risk of getting sike from her child

- Now let's jump forward in time. Click on **Leave the Floor** and then on **Restart the Program**.
- Sign in to work with Stephanie Brown during Period of Care 2.
- Click on **Go to Nurses' Station** and then on **304**.
- Click on **Patient Care** and then on **Nurse-Client Interactions**.
- Now select and view the video titled **1145: Teaching—Disease Sequelae**. (*Note*: Check the virtual clock to see whether enough time has elapsed. You can use the fast-forward feature to advance the time by 2-minute intervals if the video is not yet available. Then click again on **Patient Care** and **Nurse-Client Interactions** to refresh the screen.)

4. Discuss the most common potential sequelae associated with meningitis. Incorporate the mechanism of injury in your answer.

Extension of loccalize infection such as otitis media, sinusitis, Pharyngitis, or pneumonia in to CSF. If skin is broken & comunication b/t skin, sinuses, & CSF occure. Also may occure with a lumbar puncture, skull fracture, or surgery

meningitis can damage nerves in ear causing hearing loss

5. Is Stephanie Brown receiving any treatment or medication that may contribute to permanent injury? (*Hint:* Use the Drug Guide if needed.)

Mon
Cefotaxime IV: nephrotoxicity
baclofen PO
docusate sodium PO
Senna PO
D5.45 with 2mEq KCl/100ml (IV continuous)
Vancomycin IV: ototoxicity, nephrotoxicity

- Next, click on **Leave the Floor** and then on **Restart the Program**.
- Sign in to work with Stephanie Brown again, this time for Period of Care 3.
- Click on **Go to Nurses' Station**.
- Click on Room **304**.
- Click on **Patient Care** and then on **Nurse-Client Interactions**.
- Select and view the video titled **1510: Nurse-Patient Communication**. (*Note*: Check the virtual clock to see whether enough time has elapsed. You can use the fast-forward feature to advance the time by 2-minute intervals if the video is not yet available. Then click again on **Patient Care** and **Nurse-Client Interactions** to refresh the screen.)

6. What is the nurse's assessment and decision? Stephany reports pain

- IV site is red and has edema
- replace IV

7. The nurse explains to Stephanie Brown that she is going to apply a local anesthetic. What is a more age-appropriate way of saying this?

I'm going to apply a cream to your hand so it won't hurt

8. EMLA cream is a topical anesthetic used with children. It is applied to Intact skin and then covered with an tegaderm dressing. It should be applied 60 minutes before the procedure.

9. Notice the nurse's interaction with Stephanie and her mother. Why is Stephanie, who is only 3 years old, included in the explanation?

So that Stephanie knows what will be done and why the cream is being aplied

10. At Stephanie Brown's age, how might she perceive her hospital experience? What are some of her fears related to this experience?

- hospital experience could be scary and
- she has fear of pain

11. Notice Stephanie Brown's mother's behavior. How might that affect Stephanie's perceptions?

-her mother is calm, helping with stretches this will help Stephanie stay calm

LESSON 17

Caring for a Young Child with Cerebral Palsy

Reading Assignment: Health Promotion During Early Childhood (Chapter 7)
The Child with a Neurologic Alteration
(Chapter 52, pages 1411-1418 and 1424-1427)

Patient: Stephanie Brown, Room 304

Goal: Demonstrate an understanding of caring for a child with cerebral palsy (CP).

Objectives:

1. Describe the behaviors and problems associated with the most common types of CP.
2. Discuss a range of etiologic factors associated with CP.
3. Explain the importance of early diagnosis and treatment to the child's optimal level of function.
4. Discuss the nursing care needs of a child with CP.

Exercise 1

Virtual Hospital Activity

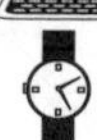

30 minutes

- Sign in to work at Pacific View Regional Hospital on the Pediatrics Floor for Period of Care 1. (*Note:* If you are already in the virtual hospital from a previous exercise, click on **Leave the Floor** and then on **Restart the Program** to get to the sign-in window.)
- From the Patient List, select Stephanie Brown.
- Click on **Get Report**.
- Click on **Go to Nurses' Station**.

1. What is CP?

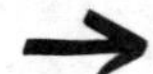

- Click on **Chart** and then on **304**.
- Click on and review the **History and Physical**.
- Click on **Return to Nurses' Station**.
- Click on **304** to go to Stephanie Brown's room.
- Click on **Patient Care** and then on **Physical Assessment**. Perform a focused assessment.

2. Based on your assessment of Stephanie Brown, list any behaviors she demonstrates that are associated with CP.

3. What might be an etiologic factor in Stephanie Brown's situation?

4. Early recognition and treatment are important to fostering achievement of optimal development. Why is CP often not diagnosed until about 2 years of age?

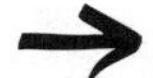

- Click on **Nurse-Client Interactions**.
- Select and view the video titled **0750: Caring for the Child with CP**. (*Note*: Check the virtual clock to see whether enough time has elapsed. You can use the fast-forward feature to advance the time by 2-minute intervals if the video is not yet available. Then click again on **Patient Care** and **Nurse-Client Interactions** to refresh the screen.)

5. What is the nurse doing as she listens to Stephanie Brown's mother explain problems Stephanie has related to CP.

6. What problem is Stephanie Brown at risk for during her hospitalization? (*Hint:* You will need to consider her developmental age.)

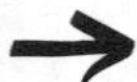

- Click on **Chart** and then on **304**.
- Click on **Nursing Admission** and review for data about Stephanie's development.

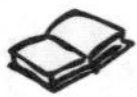

7. Assume Stephanie Brown has recently turned 3 years of age. Using the information in Chapter 7 regarding milestones for her age, determine one skill that Stephanie should have completed, one that she is working on, and one that she is not yet ready for. Do this for one of the four skill areas (gross motor, language, cognitive, fine motor, and personal/social).

Exercise 2

Virtual Hospital Activity

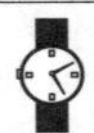

20 minutes

- Sign in to work at Pacific View Regional Hospital on the Pediatrics Floor for Period of Care 3. (*Note:* If you are already in the virtual hospital from a previous exercise, click on **Leave the Floor** and then on **Restart the Program** to get to the sign-in window.)
- From the Patient List, select Stephanie Brown.
- Click on **Get Report**.
- Click on **Go to Nurses' Station**.
- Click on **Chart** and then on **304**.
- Review Stephanie's records, in particular her **History and Physical**.

1. What type of CP does Stephanie Brown have? What are the signs that she manifests?

2. Match each type of CP with its description.

	Type	Description
_____	Spastic	a. Rigid flexor and extensor muscles; tremors
_____	Dyskinetic/athetoid	b. Increased deep tendon reflexes, hypertonia, flexion, and scissors gait
_____	Ataxic	c. Slow, writhing uncontrolled and involuntary movements
_____	Rigid	d. Loss of coordination, equilibrium, and kinesthetic sense

3. What are some aspects of a child's life on which CP can have an impact? Make sure that at least one of your answers is a psychosocial concern.

- Click on **Return to Nurses' Station**.
- Click on **304**.
- Click on **Patient Care** and then on **Nurse-Client Interactions**.
- Select and view the video titled **1530: Preventive Measures**. (*Note*: Check the virtual clock to see whether enough time has elapsed. You can use the fast-forward feature to advance the time by 2-minute intervals if the video is not yet available. Then click again on **Patient Care** and **Nurse-Client Interactions** to refresh the screen.)

4. Why does Stephanie Brown require heel cord stretching?

5. What other preventive measures have been integrated into Stephanie Brown's regimen to prevent complications associated with CP?

6. What is the nursing role with regard to supporting these endeavors?

7. Explain why nutrition is so important for the child who has CP.

Exercise 3

Writing Activity

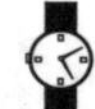

15 minutes

1. Develop a plan to teach Stephanie Brown's mother to promote self-esteem as Stephanie progresses through the stage of initiative versus guilt. First, write one or more goals.

2. Now develop nursing interventions designed to meet the goal(s) you wrote in question 1.

3. What does your community offer for children with special care needs?

4. What other local or state resources are available for these types of needs? Please include resources that would meet the needs of a wide variety of ages.

LESSON 18

Caring for a School-Age Child with Diabetes Mellitus

Reading Assignment: Health Promotion for the School-Age Child (Chapter 8)
The Child with an Endocrine or Metabolic Alteration
(Chapter 51, pages 1395-1409)

Patient: George Gonzalez, Room 301

Goal: Demonstrate an understanding of diabetes mellitus (DM) in a child, including planning care, long-term management, and teaching.

Objectives:

1. Discuss the pathophysiology of DM and diabetic ketoacidosis (DKA).
2. Compare and contrast type 1 and type 2 DM.
3. Discuss management and nursing responsibilities for insulin therapy, diet, exercise, and blood glucose monitoring.
4. Contrast causes, signs, and management of hypoglycemia and hyperglycemia.
5. Discuss the impact of growth and development on diabetes.
6. Identify learning needs of a child (and his family) newly diagnosed with diabetes.
7. Develop a plan for teaching a child independence with care of diabetes.

Exercise 1

Virtual Hospital Activity

30 minutes

- Sign in to work at Pacific View Regional Hospital on the Pediatrics Floor for Period of Care 1. (*Note:* If you are already in the virtual hospital from a previous exercise, click on **Leave the Floor** and then on **Restart the Program** to get to the sign-in window.)
- From the Patient List, select George Gonzalez.
- Click on **Go to Nurses' Station**.
- Click on **Chart** and then on **301**.
- Click on **Emergency Department** and review this record.

1. George Gonzalez has been admitted with a diagnosis of DKA. What does this mean? What are the signs of DKA?

DKA is the consequence of severe insulin deficit leading to hyperglycemia and presence of ketone bodies in the blood, followed by metabolic acidosis. Signs of DKA are: abdominal & chest pain, nausea & vomiting, fruity breath smell, decrease LOC, Kussmaul respirations and symptoms of dehydration

2. Based on the textbook and George Gonzalez's chart, what makes George at particular risk for developing diabetes?

- ↑ urine output
- high blood glucose (735)
- 11yrs 27.1kg

3. Match the following to show your understanding of the differences between type 1 and type 2 DM.

	Characteristic	Type of DM
a	This is the most common childhood endocrine disease.	a. Type 1
a	This type results from autoimmune process disorder.	b. Type 2
b	Cells are unable to use insulin.	
b	Genetic predisposition is a factor.	
a	The pancreas is unable to produce insulin.	
b	Obesity commonly coexists with this type.	

4. What was George Gonzalez's condition like when he was admitted? Was there a precipitating factor?

Blood sugar was high and complains of nausea and stomachache. Not injecting insulin consistently and eating "whatever"

5. In George's situation upon admission, what type of insulin is used and why? Identify any nursing concerns with the administration of insulin IV.

Regular insulin IV

6. What are the signs of hyperglycemia?

increased urination, increased thirst, fatigue, blurred vision, weight loss (gradual, over several weeks

7. What are the signs of hypoglycemia?

Trembling, sweating, tachycardia, pallor, clammy skin

8. For which of the following nursing diagnoses is there evidence in George Gonzalez's situation?
   a. Fluid volume deficit related to abnormal fluid losses through diuresis and emesis
   b. Risk for injury from altered acid-base balance leading to ketone production and acidosis related to lack of insulin
   c. Knowledge deficit related to unfamiliarity with home management during sick days

9. What is your rationale for your answer to question 8? Provide the data that lead you to your choice of nursing diagnosis.

- HbA_{1C} 15.2
- PH 7.25
- Urinalysis trace ketones, 4+ glucose

10. What ongoing assessments need to be made? (Focus on the admission diagnosis.)

→ • Click on **Diagnostic Reports** and review the record.

11. What is HbA_{1C}? Explain its use as a diagnostic tool. How does the normal HbA_{1C} compare with George Gonzalez's labs?

HbA_{1C} is a lab test that evaluates long-term blood glucose control by measuring glycosylation of a portion of the hemoglobin. In diabetes the HbA_{1C} is elevated.

Exercise 2

Virtual Hospital Activity

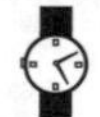

30 minutes

- Sign in to work at Pacific View Regional Hospital on the Pediatrics Floor for Period of Care 1. (*Note:* If you are already in the virtual hospital from a previous exercise, click on **Leave the Floor** and then on **Restart the Program** to get to the sign-in window.)
- From the Patient List, select George Gonzalez.
- Click on **Go to Nurses' Station**.
- Click on **301** at the bottom of the screen.
- Click on **Patient Care** and then on **Nurse-Client Interactions**.
- Select and view the video titled **0730: Supervision—Glucose Testing**. (*Note*: Check the virtual clock to see whether enough time has elapsed. You can use the fast-forward feature to advance the time by 2-minute intervals if the video is not yet available. Then click again on **Patient Care** and **Nurse-Client Interactions** to refresh the screen.)

1. What did the nurse do that facilitated George Gonzalez's honesty about his testing behavior and how he feels about it?

The nurse was calm, listned attentivley,
and validated what he was saying.

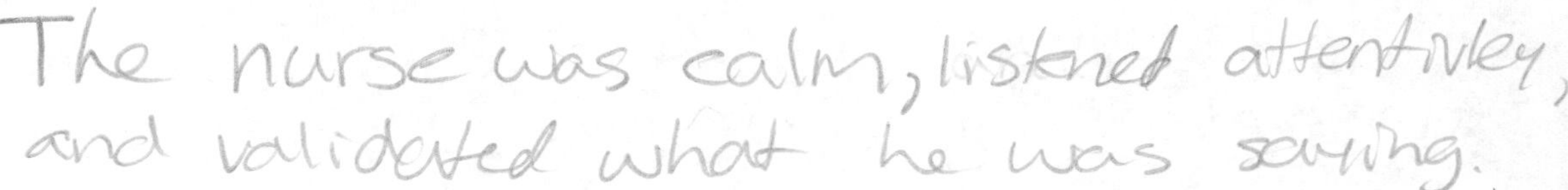

2. What is the nurse trying to accomplish when she asks George Gonzalez to do his own finger stick? How does his developmental stage affect his compliance with treatment?

The nurse wants to assess if he can do it properly.

3. What are some reasons why George Gonzalez may be noncompliant with blood glucose testing?

-he doesn't like all the needles
-he feels fine so he doesn't check it
-he doesn't have time

- Select and view the video titled **0745: Self-Administering Insulin**. (*Note*: Check the virtual clock to see whether enough time has elapsed. You can use the fast-forward feature to advance the time by 2-minute intervals if the video is not yet available. Then click again on **Patient Care** and **Nurse-Client Interactions** to refresh the screen.)

4. What does the nurse do that is positive as she observes George Gonzalez give his injection?

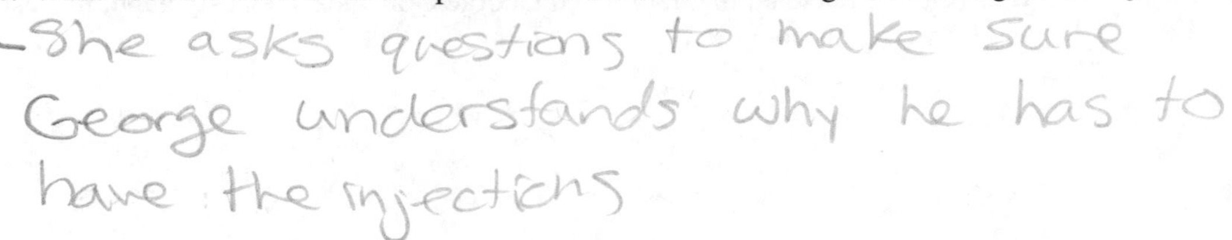
-She asks questions to make sure George understands why he has to have the injections

5. Explain the content and methods you would use in teaching the skill of self-administration of insulin.

6. What are possible barriers to learning the skill of injection technique?

7. List areas of content associated with discussing site rotations.

To decrease variations in absorption a different location ~~should~~ within a major injection site? should be used for one day

8. The abdomen is the site from which insulin is most rapidly absorbed.

George Gonzalez needs insulin. Complete the following questions before going to the Medication Room.

9. Match each type of insulin with its corresponding characteristics.

	Characteristic	Type of Insulin
a	Onset of 30-60 minutes	a. Regular; Short-acting
b	Onset of 2-4 hours	b. NPH: intermediate-acting
b	Peak at 4-10 hours	
a	Peak at 2-3 hours	30 - 1h 2-4 5-8 10-16
a	Duration of 5-8 hours	2-3 4-10
b	Duration of 10-16 hours	

10. At what point during the day is George Gonzalez most at risk for a hypoglycemic reaction?

In the middle of the night

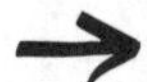

- Click on **Chart** and then on **301**.
- Click on **Physician's Orders**. Find the order for George Gonzalez's morning dose of insulin.

12 Units NPH + 6 units Lispro

11. Using George Gonzalez's morning insulin order, describe the steps for drawing up two forms of insulin in one syringe.

12. Why is the short-acting insulin always drawn up first?

Before going to the Medication Room, complete any necessary assessments.

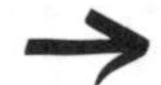

- Click on **MAR** to check the order for insulin; then click on **Return to Room 301**.
- Click on **Medication Room**.
- Using the six rights, prepare the correct dose of insulin for George Gonzalez. When you have prepared the medication, return to George's room and administer it, again following the six rights. (*Hint:* Try to perform these steps on your own. If you need help, refer to pages 26-30 and 37-41 in the **Getting Started** section of this workbook.)
- After administering the insulin, click on **Leave the Floor** and then on **Look at Your Preceptor's Evaluations**.
- Next, click on **Medication Scorecard** and review the feedback. How did you do?

Exercise 3

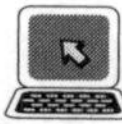

Virtual Hospital Activity

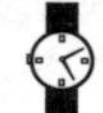

30 minutes

- Sign in to work at Pacific View Regional Hospital on the Pediatrics Floor for Period of Care 2. (*Note:* If you are already in the virtual hospital from a previous exercise, click on **Leave the Floor** and then on **Restart the Program** to get to the sign-in window.)
- From the Patient List, select George Gonzalez.
- Click on **Go to Nurses' Station** and then **301**.

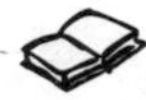

1. List the learning needs of a patient newly diagnosed with diabetes. (Consider the list provided on page 1404 in your textbook.)

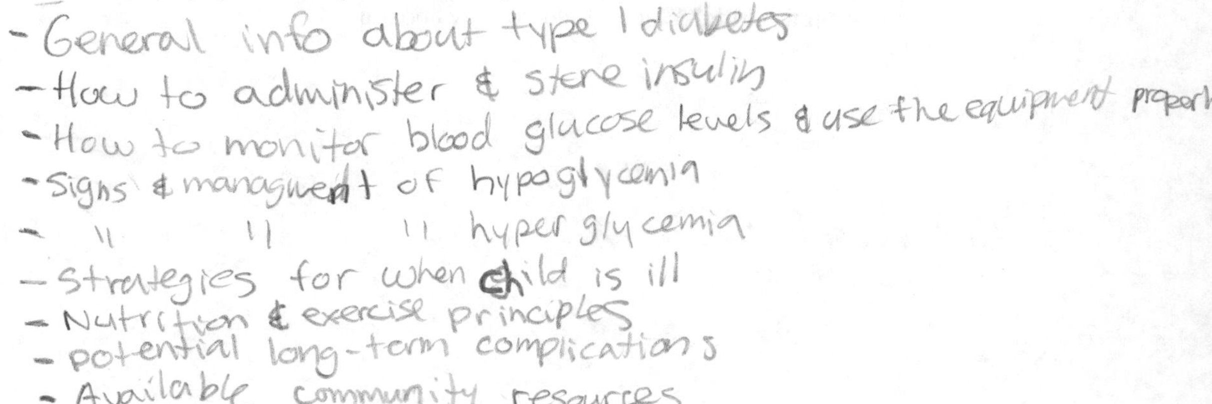

- General info about type I diabetes
- How to administer & store insulin
- How to monitor blood glucose levels & use the equipment properly
- Signs & management of hypoglycemia
- " " " hyperglycemia
- Strategies for when child is ill
- Nutrition & exercise principles
- potential long-term complications
- Available community resources

2. Which of the above learning needs apply directly to George Gonzalez and his family?

3. What anticipatory guidance can you offer George Gonzalez's mother with regard to how insulin needs change as he moves toward adolescence?

4. Discuss the relationship among insulin, food, and exercise. Explain it in terms that would be understandable for George Gonzalez and his family.

The insulin dosage is balanced with food intake, so consisten intake is important particularly carbohydrates. Exercise enhances the action of insulin in lowering blood glucose levels

5. Did you consider the "honeymoon phase" as part of your discussion? Why is this significant to parent teaching? What should you say about it?

It's important to teach parents about the honeymoon phase to avoid the misconception that the diabetes is going away. The honeymoon phase is characterized by hypoglycemia & decreased need for insulin. It can last a few weeks to a year or longer. Also it's important to recognize & treat hypoglycemia

- Click on **Patient Care** and then on **Nurse-Client Interactions**.
- Select and view the video titled **1115: Teaching—Disease Process**. (*Note*: Check the virtual clock to see whether enough time has elapsed. You can use the fast-forward feature to advance the time by 2-minute intervals if the video is not yet available. Then click again on **Patient Care** and **Nurse-Client Interactions** to refresh the screen.)

6. What are the sequelae of untreated or poorly managed diabetes? Explain why they occur.

7. Evaluate George Gonzalez's understanding of his condition and management of hypoglycemia.

8. George Gonzalez's mother seems to have a good __________ understanding.

9. Given the responses of George Gonzalez and his mother, is there a need for teaching in this area? If so, what teaching techniques would be most effective?

LESSON **19**

Caring for a Teen with an Eating Disorder

Reading Assignment: Health Promotion for the Adolescent (Chapter 9)
Psychosocial Problems in Children and Families (Chapter 53, pages 1462-1465)

Patient: Tiffany Sheldon, Room 305

Goal: Demonstrate an understanding of multidisciplinary care for a teenager with an eating disorder.

Objectives:

1. Compare and contrast the description, etiology, and typical behaviors associated with anorexia nervosa and bulimia nervosa.
2. Discuss the physiologic impact of anorexia nervosa and bulimia nervosa.
3. Discuss the multidisciplinary approach necessary for treatment of eating disorders.
4. Explore the challenges of providing nursing care for patients with anorexia nervosa or bulimia nervosa.

Exercise 1

Writing Activity

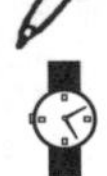

15 minutes

1. Compare and contrast anorexia and bulimia by matching each problem with its characteristics. (*Hint:* Although some behaviors may seem to overlap, they are usually associated more closely with one problem rather than the other. Choose the problem *most* closely associated with each characteristic.)

	Characteristic	Problem
a	Deliberate refusal of food to maintain body weight	a. Anorexia nervosa
b	Recurrent episodes of binging and a sense of loss of control	b. Bulimia nervosa
b	Excessive use of vomiting, laxatives, diuretics, or exercise	
a	Possible amenorrhea—both primary and secondary	
~~a~~ b	Persistent irrational concern with body weight and shape	
a	Body image that is contrary to reality	
a	Ritualistic eating pattern	
b	Binge eating and purging	
a	Muscle wasting, dull and brittle hair, lanugo	
____	Risk for fluid and electrolyte imbalance	
b	Tooth erosion	

2. Give an example of an eating pattern that might be found in a person with anorexia nervosa. What often underlies such behavior?

A person with anorexia nervosa may only eat at a certain time of day because this enhances the individual's sense of control over food intake.

3. How is it believed that family function and culture play into the problem of eating disorders?

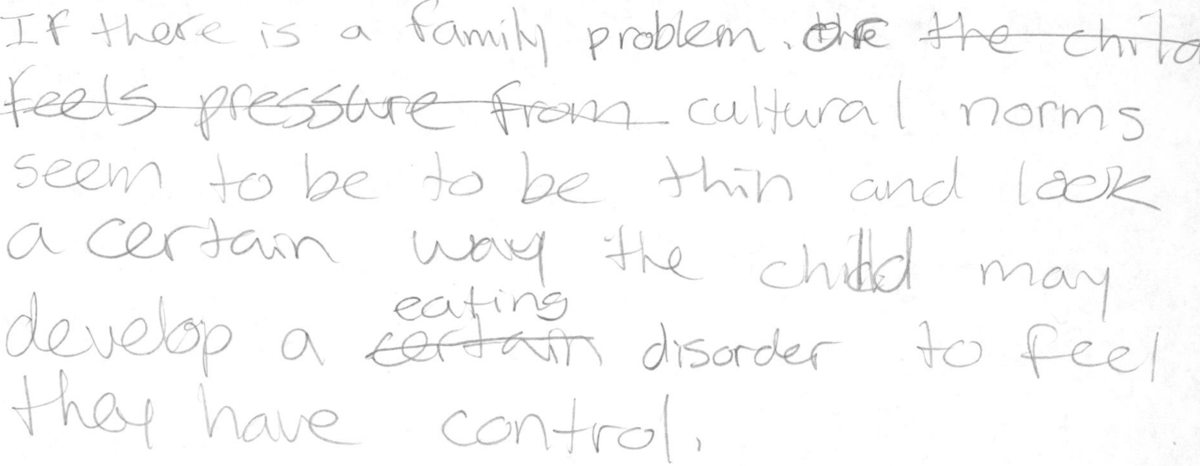

4. What are some secondary gains achieved through eating disorders? (*Hint:* Secondary gains are indirect "benefits" that the patient gets from having his or her disease.)

Exercise 2

Virtual Hospital Activity

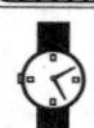

30 minutes

- Sign in to work at Pacific View Regional Hospital on the Pediatrics Floor for Period of Care 1. (*Note:* If you are already in the virtual hospital from a previous exercise, click on **Leave the Floor** and then on **Restart the Program** to get to the sign-in window.)
- From the Patient List, select Tiffany Sheldon.
- Click on **Go to Nurses' Station**.
- Click on **Chart** and then on **305**.
- Review the **Nursing Admission** and the **History and Physical**.

1. What in Tiffany Sheldon's history is indicative of her diagnosis of anorexia nervosa?

-Parent's divorced 3 years ago and both parents remarried

2. Did you identify the family crisis (divorce of parents) as a precipitating factor in Tiffany Sheldon's situation? Did you include the fact that she is an "A" student in your list? Why should you see these factors as red flags?

- Click on **Return to Nurses' Station**.
- Click on Room **305** at the bottom of the screen.
- Click on **Patient Care**.
- Complete a head-to-toe assessment, watching for assessment data that are consistent with anorexia nervosa.

3. As you complete your assessment, what stands out to you? How much does nutritional status affect the total patient?

- Decreased sub q tissue
- Dry oral mucosa
- Poor skin turgor
- Hair thin & dry with random areas of alopecia visible
- Withdrawn & listless with flat affect
- heart rate 44 bpm and irregular
- Decreased muscle tone & impaired strength
- Brittle nails
- Decreased activity level
- Unsteady & slow gait

- Click on **Nurse-Client Interactions**.
- Select and view the video titled **0730: Initial Assessment**. (*Note*: Check the virtual clock to see whether enough time has elapsed. You can use the fast-forward feature to advance the time by 2-minute intervals if the video is not yet available. Then click again on **Patient Care** and **Nurse-Client Interactions** to refresh the screen.)

4. Tiffany Sheldon has been described as having a flat affect, being withdrawn, and avoiding eye contact. How would you describe her behavior at the time of this interaction?

- She maintained eye contact
- She would respond apropriately when asked questions

5. What is the most effective communication to use with Tiffany Sheldon?

written communication with oral explanation

6. In addition to nursing assessment, what multidimensional assessments and interventions are important to developing an appropriate plan of care for Tiffany?

7. How do you think Tiffany Sheldon might respond to being told that she will be seen by an Eating Disorders Team?

Tiffany has been seen by an eating disorders team before.

8. What is the nurse's role in identifying and/or coordinating care and services that Tiffany Sheldon requires during her inpatient stay?

Exercise 3

Virtual Hospital Activity

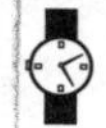

45 minutes

The first order of business with a patient who has anorexia nervosa is to correct any imbalances. Keep this in mind as you work through this exercise.

- Sign in to work at Pacific View Regional Hospital on the Pediatrics Floor for Period of Care 1. (*Note:* If you are already in the virtual hospital from a previous exercise, click on **Leave the Floor** and then on **Restart the Program** to get to the sign-in window.)
- From the Patient List, select Tiffany Sheldon.
- Click on **Go to Nurses' Station**.
- Click on **Chart** and then on **305**.
- Review the chart, especially the **Physician's Orders** and the **Laboratory Reports**.

1. What is being done to assess for and manage Tiffany Sheldon's fluid and electrolyte imbalance?

Labs: - Chem 7, BUN, creatinine, & glucose q4h
- Phosphorus, calcium, magnesium q8h

Strict intake & output

2. What do Tiffany Sheldon's lab results tell you about her fluid and electrolyte status? Report on the ones that give you specific information.

3. Tiffany Sheldon did not have a pH level done. A patient with anorexia nervosa is at risk for metabolic alkalosis. What would happen to the pH in this instance?

4. List the objective assessment data that indicate Tiffany Sheldon is dehydrated.

-Voids only twice a day small amount
-Dry mucosa
-Poor skin colour

5. Why is Tiffany Sheldon on a cardiac monitor?

6. Tiffany Sheldon is receiving IV fluid with potassium chloride added. What is the order? What are the nursing responsibilities before and during potassium administration?

IV fluids with D5.45 at 80mL/hr. Add 20mEq KCl/L to IV when paitent voids

7. a. Identify a generic nursing diagnosis for hydration problems in patients with anorexia nervosa.

   b. Now rewrite this nursing diagnosis so that it accurately reflects Tiffany's situation.

Next, begin thinking about how adequate caloric intake is achieved.

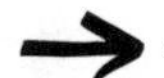

- Click on **Return to Nurse's Station** and then on **Leave the Floor**.
- From the Floor Menu, select **Restart the Program**.
- Sign in to work at Pacific View Regional Hospital on the Pediatrics Floor for Period of Care 2.
- From the Patient List, select Tiffany Sheldon.
- Click on **Go to Nurses' Station** and then on **305** at the bottom of the screen.
- Click on **Patient Care** and then on **Nurse-Client Interactions**.
- Select and view the video titled **1115: Managing Anorexia Nervosa**. (*Note*: Check the virtual clock to see whether enough time has elapsed. You can use the fast-forward feature to advance the time by 2-minute intervals if the video is not yet available. Then click again on **Patient Care** and **Nurse-Client Interactions** to refresh the screen.)

8. Discuss the cultural beliefs and personal perceptions that influence the development of eating disorders. Consider both males and females in your discussion.

9. What is the value of an eating contract for Tiffany Sheldon?

- Meet target calories & weight gain

10. What is the rationale for the diet orders that are part of the eating contract?

- liquid supplements
- gradually ↑ calories
- No exercise
- No diet pills, laxitives, self induced vomiting

11. The eating contract specifies 2100 calories per day to facilitate weight gain.

12. What supportive interventions might the nurse provide to help Tiffany Sheldon remain compliant?

- Ask what favorit foods are

Now, consider the emotional aspects of Tiffany Sheldon's care.

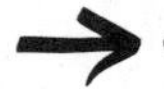

- Click on **Leave the Floor** and then on **Restart the Program**.
- Sign in to work at Pacific View Regional Hospital on the Pediatrics Floor for Period of Care 3.
- From the Patient List, select Tiffany Sheldon.
- Click on **Go to Nurses' Station**.
- Click on **305** at the bottom of the screen.
- Click on **Patient Care** and then on **Nurse-Client Interactions**.
- Select and view the video titled **1500: Relapse—Contributing Factors**. (*Note*: Check the virtual clock to see whether enough time has elapsed. You can use the fast-forward feature to advance the time by 2-minute intervals if the video is not yet available. Then click again on **Patient Care** and **Nurse-Client Interactions** to refresh the screen.)

13. What does Tiffany Sheldon say about what has caused her relapse? What recent events, if any, may have contributed to her having an acute episode of her anorexia nervosa?

-Dad
-Divorce

14. What did the psychiatrist do to effectively elicit Tiffany Sheldon's concerns?

-Spent time alone

15. What multidimensional factors will contribute to Tiffany Sheldon's ability to comply with the eating contract that has been developed? What barriers may be present?

-She feels it's to much food to eat

16. A patient with an eating disorder may not like the sensations associated with refeeding. Develop strategies to help Tiffany Sheldon overcome barriers to the success of her eating disorder plan.

~~School~~

17. School nurses or nurses in community settings may play several roles with teens who have anorexia nervosa. Discuss one of the primary roles.

School nurses can organize awareness programs, which offer opportunities for inquiries from children who might not normally speak about their eating problems or concerns about weight.

LESSON 20

Caring for a Child and Family in the Emergency Department

Reading Assignment: Emergency Care of the Child
(Chapter 34, pages 841-850 and 857-861)
The Child with a Neurologic Alteration
(Chapter 52, pages 1411-1421 and 1426-1430)

Patient: Tommy Douglas, Room 302

Goal: Demonstrate an understanding of the needs and care for a child and family experiencing an emergency.

Objectives:

1. Identify factors that may culminate in a stressful environment in the Emergency Department.
2. Discuss nursing interventions supportive to the child and family who are in the Emergency Department.
3. Discuss the concept of "across the room" assessment and priority setting for a child in the Emergency Department.
4. Explore the implications of growth and development in emergency care.
5. Explore medications frequently used in traumatic emergency situations.
6. Identify priority concerns related to head injury.

Exercise 1

Writing Activity

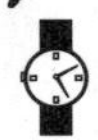

20 minutes

1. List and explain five or six factors that can contribute to creating a stressful environment when a child is brought to the Emergency Department after a traumatic event.

- fears children have at various developmental stage (ex. separation, pain, altered body image)
- fear of the unknowen
- Unfamiliar with setting, the staff, the equipment, & procedures
- Parents are unsure which increases childs stress
- Not knowing what is going on.

2. For each of the factors you listed above, develop a nursing intervention to minimize stress. If you have had experience in such an environment (even during an observation), you have an opportunity to be creative here.

- Communicate an attitude of calm confidence
- Establish a trusting relationship with child & family
- Encourage care givers to stay with child when appropriate
- Explain procedure to both the child & parent in 'normal' language

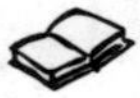

3. Review the general guidelines covered on pages 841-843 in your textbook. How many of them did you incorporate in your intervention list? For any interventions you listed that are not in the textbook, consider how easy or realistic they would be to implement. Write a reflective comment.

4. The priority assessment on a new admission is ____________________.

5. What is meant by the notion of "assessment from across the room"? Identify some assessments that can be made in this manner.

6. Rank the following care items in order of priority by numbering from 1 (highest priority) to 7 (lowest priority).

Care Item	Priority Ranking
Trauma scoring	
Assessment of child's coping	
Circulatory assessment	
History of injury	
Breathing assessment	
Airway assessment	
Signs of other injury	

7. Choose two age groups of children that you would find especially challenging to work with in the Emergency Department. For each age group, explain the challenges and share a nursing intervention to help.

Addescent

- may exaggerate or underplay the seriousness of a condition
- believe their point of view is always right

Nursing intervention explain procedures or treatment carefully and allow time for questions

Toddler

- they don't respond well to restrictions
- they like to push any limits imposed

Nursing intervention: Give praise & distractions to increase cooperation

Parents and caregivers need a great deal of support. Nurses need to be able to anticipate fears and anxieties in order to craft careful communication to elicit and respond to concerns.

8. What are the three greatest fears parents have when their child is brought to the Emergency Department?

9. Parents may feel pushed aside in the Emergency Department. How can the nurse deal with this problem?

Exercise 2

Virtual Hospital Activity

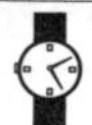

45 minutes

- Sign in to work at Pacific View Regional Hospital on the Pediatrics Floor for Period of Care 1. (*Note:* If you are already in the virtual hospital from a previous exercise, click on **Leave the Floor** and then on **Restart the Program** to get to the sign-in window.)
- From the Patient List, select Tommy Douglas.
- Click on **Go to Nurses' Station**.
- Click on **Chart** and then on **302**.
- Review Tommy Douglas' chart, especially the **Emergency Department** and **Physician's Orders** sections.

1. Describe the circumstances of Tommy Douglas' admission. Include such information as the nature of his injury and the people around him.

2. Explain what is meant by blunt trauma.

3. Explain the mechanism of the acceleration-deceleration injury that occurs with a major head injury.

The shearing force of the initial impact moves the brain forward, followed by a countering backward movement of the brain in the skull. Shearing force produces bruising, tearing, and bleeding

4. What are the priorities for initial management of a head injury?

5. A child with a head injury is at risk for ______________________________ and ______________________.

6. List the signs of increased intracranial pressure based on Tommy Douglas' developmental level.

7. Review Tommy Douglas' initial medication orders (from admission on Tuesday through Wednesday morning). List the medications ordered and give a reason for each order.

- Click on **Return to Nurses' Station**.
- Click on the **Drug** icon in the lower left corner of the screen.
- Review the medications ordered for Tommy, looking for any information you need to administer them.

8. Do you see any concerns? Explain.

Select one of the medications that need to be administered during this period of care and complete the following steps to prepare and administer it.

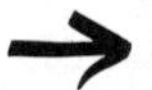

- Click on **Return to Nurses' Station** and then on **Medication Room**.
- Using the six rights, select, prepare, and administer the medication to be given. When you have finished the preparation, return to Tommy's room and administer the medication. (*Hint:* Although you should be getting more comfortable with the steps of preparing and administering medications, you can refer to pages 26-30 and 37-41 in the **Getting Started** section if you need help.)
- To obtain feedback, click on **Leave the Floor**.
- Click on **Look at Your Preceptor's Evaluations** and then on **Medication Scorecard**.

9. Review the feedback on your Medication Scorecard. Are there any areas in which you need to make changes? If so, select another medication ordered for Tommy and practice the procedure again.

- To return to the Pediatrics Floor, click on **Return to Evaluations**, **Return to Menu**, and **Restart the Program**.
- Sign in again to work with Tommy Douglas during Period of Care 1.
- Click on **Go to Nurses' Station**.
- Click on **Chart** and then on **302**.
- Click on **Physician's Orders**.

10. $NaHCO_3$ is ordered to be given STAT. How much time do you have to prepare and administer the medication?

11. Why is Tommy Douglas receiving bolus infusions?

- Click on **Nursing Admission** and review.

12. The physician has ordered a rate increase for norepinephrine. The drug was running at a rate of _______________. It has been increased to a rate of _______________. (*Hint:* Find Tommy's weight in the Nursing Admission to do the necessary calculations.)

- Now click on the **Emergency Department** tab and search the record for neurologic assessment data.

13. What significant neurologic data did you find in Tommy's Emergency Department record?

14. The purpose of the cerebral perfusion scan is to ________________________________.

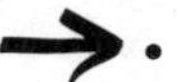

- Click on **Return to Nurses' Station**.
- Click on Room **302** at the bottom of the screen.
- Click on **Patient Care**.
- Complete a focused neurologic assessment of Tommy and then chart your findings in the EPR. (*Hint:* If you need help entering data in the EPR, refer to pages 15-16 in the **Getting Started** section of this workbook.)
- To obtain feedback, click on **Leave the Floor** and then on **Look at Your Preceptor's Evaluations**.
- Select **Examination Report** and review your evaluation.

15. Complete a narrative note related to the data compiled from the focused neurologic assessment.

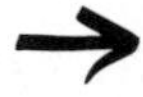

- To return to the Pediatrics Floor, click on **Return to Evaluations**, **Return to Menu**, and **Restart the Program**.
- Sign in again to work with Tommy Douglas for Period of Care 1.
- Click on **Go to Nurses' Station**.
- Click on **302** to go to Tommy Douglas' room.
- Click on **Patient Care** and then on **Nurse-Client Interactions**.
- Select and view the video titled **0730: Assessment—Neurological**. (*Note*: Check the virtual clock to see whether enough time has elapsed. You can use the fast-forward feature to advance the time by 2-minute intervals if the video is not yet available. Then click again on **Patient Care** and **Nurse-Client Interactions** to refresh the screen.)

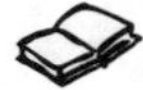

16. Describe the Glasgow Coma Scale (GCS). Include the parameters that are assessed when it is used, particularly for children. (*Hint:* Review Table 52-1 in your textbook.)

17. What was Tommy Douglas' GCS score?

18. How would you explain to Tommy's parents what the ventilator is doing?

19. Tommy's blood pressure is low. Explain why fluids help to maintain blood pressure.

LESSON 21

Providing Support for Families Experiencing the Loss of a Child

Reading Assignment: The Child with a Chronic Condition or Terminal Illness (Chapter 36)

Patient: Tommy Douglas, Room 302

Goal: Demonstrate an understanding of end-of-life care issues in the hospital setting.

Objectives:

1. Explore the range of reactions that may occur when parents are told there is no hope of saving their child's life.
2. Discuss the role of hospital ethics committees.
3. Discuss nursing responsibilities associated with organ donation.
4. Discuss the concept of "allowing" a child to die.
5. Identify strategies to support parents and children as a child dies.

Exercise 1

Virtual Hospital Activity

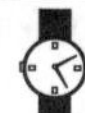

30 minutes

- Sign in to work at Pacific View Regional Hospital on the Pediatrics Floor for Period of Care 2. (*Note:* If you are already in the virtual hospital from a previous exercise, click on **Leave the Floor** and then on **Restart the Program** to get to the sign-in window.)
- From the Patient List, select Tommy Douglas.
- Click on **Go to Nurses' Station**.
- Click on **302** at the bottom of the screen.
- Click on **Patient Care** and then on **Nurse-Client Interactions**.
- Select and view the video titled **1115: The Family (Care) Conference**. (*Note*: Check the virtual clock to see whether enough time has elapsed. You can use the fast-forward feature to advance the time by 2-minute intervals if the video is not yet available. Then click again on **Patient Care** and **Nurse-Client Interactions** to refresh the screen.)

1. Tommy Douglas has been certified as "brain dead," and a family conference has been held to inform his parents that he will not be helped by further intervention. Who are the usual participants in such a conference? What does each person bring to the discussion?

2. What is the role of the institutional ethics committee with respect to any potential conflicts in care delivery?

3. What intervention can the nurse provide to the parents after the family conference?

4. Assume that Tommy Douglas' family wants him to live "at all costs." How would you feel about this? What might be your response to Tommy's parents?

5. As Tommy Douglas' parents agree to organ donation, is there evidence of progression with anticipatory grieving?

→ • Click on **Chart** and then on **302**.
• Click on **Physician's Orders** and review.

6. Discuss the kind of care that is being provided for Tommy Douglas during this time.

7. Tommy Douglas is receiving hospice care. Contrast palliative and hospice care.

Let's check in on Tommy Douglas' family a little later in the day.

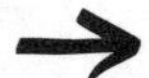

- Click on **Leave the Floor** and then on **Restart the Program**.
- Sign in to care for Tommy Douglas, this time during Period of Care 3.
- Click on **Go to Nurses' Station** and then on **302** at the bottom of the screen.
- Click on **Patient Care** and then on **Nurse-Client Interactions**.
- Select and view the video titled **1500: Nurse-Family Communication**. (*Note*: Check the virtual clock to see whether enough time has elapsed. You can use the fast-forward feature to advance the time by 2-minute intervals if the video is not yet available. Then click again on **Patient Care** and **Nurse-Client Interactions** to refresh the screen.)

8. Evaluate the nurse's approach in dealing with a family in crisis. Did the nurse demonstrate empathy? If so, how?

9. Is the nurse's body language congruent with his verbal communication?

Exercise 2

Writing Activity

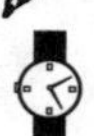

30 minutes

"Allowing" a child to die is a very difficult concept. Parents go through several stages as their child dies.

1. Discuss what parents go through when their child experiences a life-threatening injury or illness that then becomes terminal.

2. Parents frequently need to talk about what is happening while their child is dying. Why?

3. What anticipatory guidance would you offer grieving parents for dealing with other children in their family?

4. What information needs to be provided about the dying process?

5. How might you guide parents at the time of death? (*Hint:* Remember that allowing a child to die is tremendously difficult for parents.)

6. How are siblings of a dying child likely to view death?

7. How would you provide care for the family members after their child's death?

8. Assume that you enter the room and find the parents sobbing as they sit with their dying child. Does this mean you have not been effective with your teaching and care? What can you do for these parents?

9. What do you think the concept of "chronic sorrow" means?

10. Discuss ways that nurses who care for dying children cope with their own grief.